THE
HEALTHY
HEDONIST

A FUN LOVER'S GUIDE
TO GREAT HEALTH

JANET
BRIDGERS

Published by Terracotta Books & Media
Oxnard, California
Copyright 2002 Janet Bridgers

Published by: Terracotta Books & Media
716 N. Ventura Rd. #375, Oxnard, CA 93030 U.S.A.
thehealthyhedonist.com

This book is for informational and educational purposes only. The
author is a health researcher. The material in this book is not
meant to replace qualified advice with regard to your specific
healthcare needs. Never change any treatment or medication
without consulting with your physician. Though the book lends
itself to self-help, either you, or the physician who examines and
treats you, must take the responsibility for the uses made of this
book. The author and Terracotta Books & Media do not take the
medical or legal responsibility of having the contents herein
considered appropriate to all individuals. Because each person is
different, it is strongly suggested that you consult with a health
practitioner familiar with the information if aspects of this
program constitute a significant change from your current
lifestyle and behaviors.

First Printing 2002   ISBN 0-9714921-9-0
Library of Congress Control Number: 2002094322

Cover Design: Roger Merrill, Missoula, Montana
Interior Design: Roger Merrill & Casa Graphics, Burbank, CA
Edited by Robin Quinn, quinnrobin@aol.com

Printed in the United States of America.
Text on 60# recycled offset by Badger, 30% Post Consumer Waste.
Cover printed on C1S Cornwall Coated by Domtar, 15% PCW.
Type: Jansen

DEDICATION

I dedicate this book to three men.
First, to my father, Frank H. Bridgers, whose contributions
to my life are inestimable, and whose love and
warm sense of humor I will always treasure.
It's also dedicated to the memories of William R. Buckley
and Judge Santiago E. Campos, both of Santa Fe, New Mexico.
Together, these three men consistently demonstrated how honor and
integrity could be combined with great zest for life.

"Too much of a good thing is wonderful."

Mae West

Contents

Part One / The Concept

Welcome to the Banquet! 13

Chapter 1. Gambling on Health? 17
How a familiar card game helps explain the concept of healthy hedonism.

Chapter 2. The Dry Well 23
Besides improving your social life, there are other reasons why healthy hedonism could be very important to you.

Chapter 3. The Lost Key 27
An understanding of what long-term hedonism really means produces the missing key in preventive healthcare information.

Chapter 4. Pillars of Healthy Hedonism 35
Healthy hedonism is not only supported by science, but by thousands of years of philosophy. But don't let that put you off!

Part Two / Week-long Pleasures

Chapter 5. Wake Me Gently, Please 47
New ideas on how to take the adrenaline rush out of your early morning routine.

Chapter 6. Fruit, Nature's Fast Food 51
Fruit is all pleasure, no pain, with numerous underrated benefits. Not the least of these benefits is bold sensuality. What a nice way to start the day!

Chapter 7. Walk, Walk, Walk—Around the Block 61
The "ugly duckling" of exercise proves to be America's favorite. It's easy to implement, effective, affordable and simply civilized.

Chapter 8. Better Showering: Making the Most of a Good Thing 71
Discover a surprisingly simple one-minute investment in skin tone and great health. Find out how hot water can help loosen your back.

Chapter 9. Rediscovering Energy 79
Timing when you eat certain foods can dramatically improve your energy levels and general health. It may assist you in losing weight.

Chapter 10. Easy Exits 89
A bit of planning can reduce your exit time, as well as your morning stress.

Chapter 11. Work in Balance 95
It may not be easy to find "balance" at work. That doesn't mean it's impossible. Here are ways to approach it.

Chapter 12. Home, James! 113
Begin to relax while you drive home. Arrive in a better state of mind to enjoy your evening, your time.

Chapter 13. Tasty, Right-Fat Snacks 119
New ideas, and a few old favorites, for those times when you need a munch, plus an explanation of what "right-fat" means.

Chapter 14. Mood-Altering Strategies 133
Wholesome, legal, non-addictive and non-fattening ways to turn your home into a pleasure palace.

Chapter 15. Gifts of the Magi, Gifts for You 141
Using scents to pleasantly adjust the quality of your life at home and away.

Chapter 16. The New Art of Bathing 153
Bathing offers luxury at a price you can't afford to miss. Now it can also deliver significant health benefits.

Chapter 17. A Time of Peace 165
A few minutes to yourself before bed may be the best investment you can make in sound sleep and peace of mind.

Chapter 18. Sleep, Blissful Sleep 177
To feel good, look good, and perform well, nothing beats a good night's rest. Here's how to sleep better every night.

Part Three / Weekend Pleasures

Chapter 19. Good, Better, Best Weekends 199
Making the best days of the week even more pleasurable and productive.

Chapter 20. Juicing & Saturday Salads 207
Juicing lets you unleash your creativity and inhibitions. No time to make great salads on weekdays? Make one on Saturday to last two days!

Chapter 21. Cooking with Family & Friends 215
Ideas for great fun, great food and a headstart on mid-week meals.

Chapter 22. Eating Out & Traveling 223
Keeping the fun in those experiences that are supposed to be fun.

Chapter 23. Maximum Fun, Minimal Damage 237
How to "party hearty" with no regrets the next morning.

Chapter 24. Quality, Not Quantity 247
Finding satisfaction in the small intense experience—discovering you don't have to be wealthy to be rich.

Part Four / Weekends Just for You

Chapter 25. Detox Weekends 253
Simple, gentle and pleasurable ways to do "detox" at home.

Chapter 26. Yoga & T'ai Chi 275
How to create the feeling of a two-week vacation in just an hour and a half, while getting rid of low-back pain, stiffness and stress.

Chapter 27. Bodywork Feels Sooo Good! 285
You don't have to be ill to benefit from the most popular form of alternative medicine. And good news! Some of it you can do for yourself and others.

Chapter 28. Spa Culture without Big Bucks 295
Affordable, convenient ways to bring spa luxury to your life.

On Moving Forward 307
Every day, in every way, we're getting better and better. Really!

Part Five / More Help for You

Notes 313
I didn't make all this up.

Resources 318
Where to go for more information.

JB's Simple, Easy, Healthy and Yummy Recipes 331
Including energy bars, plus some great soup and bean recipes.

Index 341

Author's Biography 355

ACKNOWLEDGMENTS

This book would never have been accomplished without the support, encouragement and contributions of many people, including Julie Andelman, Annette Annechild, Debbie Baker, the entire Bridgers family, especially my sister Lynn Bridgers, Yvonne Burge, Bob Carr, Frank Cordell, Kelly Cosandaey, Candi Dougal, Bill Frank, Lorilee Friedland, Jane Gabrilove, Greg Godek, Ellen Stern Harris, Willy Holst, Suzanne Horner, Shar Kanan, Susan Kendrick, Dagmar King, Karen Koster, Catherine Leach, Gary Lewis, Will Maguire, Roger Merrill, Melissa Metcalfe, N.D., Suzy Milstead, Joseph Nathanson, Donna Nelson, Dan Poynter, Robin Quinn, Garth Schaefer, Selacia, Victor Sykes, Dottie Walters, Ernie and Patty Weckbaugh, Paul Williams and Irwin Zucker. Special thanks go to my husband Patrick Wall who patiently endured the ups and downs of the book-writing process and contributed great editing before the book was done. Lastly, thanks to our dogs, Bo and Boogie, who supplied comic relief and unflagging enthusiasm for walks.

See what you've done! (It's absolutely true that I couldn't have done it without you.)

Part One

The Concept

"Healthy hedonism is a way of being healthy that respects your need to relax and have a good time. Too many health concepts want to take away the pleasures you have in life, not add to them."

Welcome to the Banquet!

Come on in! I'm glad you're here.

There's a banquet table set up inside for us to enjoy together. But first, I'd like to give you a quick "tour." Then you'll have a better idea of how this party came together.

The concept of healthy hedonism isn't new. I observed it, tried it, and watched while scientific research substantiated the various elements.

Eventually I decided to write about my observations and experiences. Why? Because I didn't like the notion conveyed by many health books that healthy behavior has to be an "all or nothing" proposition. I flat-out reject *that* idea as unhealthy.

Healthy hedonism is a way of being healthy that respects your need to relax and have a good time. Too many health concepts want to take away the pleasures you have in life, not add to them. The experts who suggest them use words like "should," "must" and "never," likely causing you to experience that nasty emotion called guilt if you can't follow the regime perfectly. I say, "To hell with that!" Life's too short. Based on my understanding of the Big Picture, I believe that part of our mission here on Earth is to enjoy and celebrate life.

This is an approach to health based on pleasure. It's a very sound approach. Why? Because if you derive immediate gratification from an activity, you'll be more interested in continuing to do it, again and again. Granted, we don't all take the same degree of pleasure in the same activities, but that's what a banquet table is all about. There's something here for everyone. So try a little of this and a little of that, and go back for seconds on whatever you find here you like.

We've all become very busy, and often we have a lot of stress. If you're pressed for time in the first place, why would you want to follow a health regime that takes up enormous amounts of time, money and energy? That sounds like more stress. Healthy hedonism works easily within a busy schedule.

How did this come together? My understanding of a healthy and pleasurable approach to life began when I was growing up in New Mexico, a beautiful place that opens to the majesty of the heavens. It has a rich and diverse culture, fabulous food, lots of artists and craftspeople, and more than a few bright engineers and scientists. It's laid-back. There was time in New Mexico to enjoy friends and family, as well as the great physical beauty of the land.

I've always loved New Mexico, but California beckoned. I wanted to be part of this brewpot of contemporary culture that we call Southern California. I moved to West Hollywood where, for almost 15 years, I lived a bohemian existence in a bungalow a block below Sunset Boulevard.

I was close enough to observe how the rich and famous live. Not being gifted as an entertainer, I worked around the periphery of the music and media worlds without envy. I knew I had more genuine friendships and fewer worries than the people who lived in those big houses in the hills.

Over a long period of time, I could see a pattern emerge. Actors and actresses have ample opportunities to party and indulge. However, if they lose control, they're often out of a job. The smart ones learn how to engage in social activities, an essential part of their world, without killing their prospects for further work. As an example, I have a wonderful and beautiful friend who worked internationally as a cabaret dancer. Her bosses staged "bikini" tests where dancers were required to go onstage in bikinis, without notice. If the bosses thought that a dancer had gained a pound or two, she was out of a job with no recourse. Talk about pressure in the diet department! My friend knew every trick for eating well without gaining weight. I learned a lot from her.

Over the years, I deduced that most entertainers have a full-time job just doing the things that keep them looking good. They spend enormous amounts of time, energy and money on cosmetic surgery, tanning salons, spas, fitness trainers, massage and every beauty treatment imaginable. I didn't have the same pressure to look good that they have, and I certainly didn't make their kind of money. Still I'm vain and not ashamed to admit it. Gradually, I figured out a lot of ways to look good that don't cost much. There are tips scattered throughout the book that I've gathered as a result of being close to, if not a part of, what is known as Hollywood.

Two other major aspects of my life came together during the time I lived in West Hollywood. I became an environmentalist, and this increased my understanding of our relationship with the physical world. Later, those experiences gave me important insights into our "personal ecology."

I also began taking yoga classes at a modest, traditional yoga school off Sunset Boulevard. Yoga has been a major factor in helping me to reduce stress and develop my own sense of spiritual connectedness.

But I never stopped enjoying a good time. I've always considered margaritas to be just as important as a good stretch. There's a place on Sunset Boulevard (not far from the yoga school) that serves flaming strawberry margaritas. My personal record was four in one night, which brought me very close to my limit. Now I only drink two. Then I eat lots of enchiladas and beans. And drink lots of water. And take my vitamins. And drink dandelion tea.

I haven't changed much over the years. In many ways, I'm still a kid. Like any kid, I am always testing my limits. You can read more about the results of my personal research in Chapter 23, "Maximum Fun, Minimal Damage."

Now that you have these insights into a few of the experiences that revealed healthy hedonism to me, I invite you to help yourself to the goodies!

"We want to eat well and be entertained often. However, if the food we eat and what we do to enjoy life end up making us miserable and unhealthy, we've defeated our purpose."

Chapter One

GAMBLING ON HEALTH?

A brief review of the card game known as Blackjack, or "21," provides a good analogy for understanding the premise of *The Healthy Hedonist*.

In the game, the gambler's goal is to end up with a card count closer to 21 than the dealer's hand. Initially, two cards are dealt. After seeing the total of these first two cards, a player may ask for additional cards to try to get closer to 21. However, once the player's cards add up to more than 21, the player has lost.

There's more to Blackjack, of course, but I have simplified it to explain the following analogy.

Most of us want to make our life as pleasurable as possible. We want to eat well and be entertained often. However, if the food we eat and what we do to enjoy life end up making us miserable and unhealthy, we've defeated our purpose. We've asked for too many "cards" too often. Disability and chronic illness are the opposite of enjoyment, and if our lifestyle is leading us in that direction, we would be wise to change before our health falls apart. The trick is to learn to stay healthy without missing the party.

THE SEARCH FOR A STRATEGY

Developing a winning strategy—a happy, healthy strategy—isn't easy. There is a lot of conflicting information. Every week, medical researchers publish contradictory studies.

Finding someone to help us sift through this information is difficult. Doctors now spend roughly 15 minutes on each patient visit. Getting to know their patients as people is a luxury most doctors can't afford. Very few of them have time to act as counselors, and very few understand preventive healthcare measures such as nutrition.

A doctor, seeing that we have gained weight, is likely to say, "You need to lose weight." Or "You need to get more exercise." But then we are handed a brochure telling us pretty much what we already know, rather than receiving the personal touch of help in figuring out how to change. We most often have to do that on our own.

If you're like me and almost everyone else I know, the aspiration to make an improvement in my life, the knowledge of how to do it, and the discipline to carry it out are all very different things.

More than half the people in this country are overweight, even while slimness is glorified by our media culture. Who wants to be overweight? No one I know. If losing weight were as easy as just wanting to lose weight, there would be a lot fewer overweight people, and a lot of companies that "feed" on our desire to be slim would go out of business.

And what about the advice we get from holistic practitioners? Unfortunately, too often the holistic approach to health, if applied to the analogy of Blackjack, would be to never take a third card. Sure, such a strategy is going to win a few hands, but it's a very boring way to play Blackjack.

Holistic practitioners ask us to give up many things we might enjoy, such as coffee, sugar, alcohol, meat, dairy and wheat. It seems like they're not only asking us to totally opt out of enjoying these foods and beverages, but to opt out of what most would consider a social life as well. Avoiding all the "no-no's" in restaurants or in the course of a friend's home-cooked meal can be frustrating, if not impossible. Abiding by strict dietary constraints can make us appear difficult to our companions. Our hosts may feel, after all their work to prepare for guests, a sense of failure for not accommodating our dietary preferences, causing discomfort for the whole gathering.

Many holistic health practitioners, in my experience, naturally enjoy a rather ascetic lifestyle. I know such a person intimately, because I'm married to him, a man of awesome willpower. If my husband says he's going to stop doing something that's damaging to his health, he just does it; he stops cold turkey.

I'm not like that. I love wine and an occasional beer. I'm addicted to caffeine. I think rice pasta has a lousy texture compared to wheat pasta. And what would life be without a little bit of chocolate?

Don't get me wrong. I believe wholeheartedly in the power of natural and holistic healthcare. I've known its benefits for a long time, and now am more informed about them than ever. Several people very close to me have severe dietary restrictions, necessitated not only by the need to recover a measure of health, but also to literally stay alive. Still each of them has found ways, despite these sacrifices, to enrich their lives. Their pain and suffering has been so much lessened that there's no question that such changes are worthwhile. Knowing these people, and experiencing their joys and tribulations, has proven to me beyond question that a whole-foods diet, nutritional supplements and insightful healthcare (some of it alternative, some of it mainstream) can produce miracles. These friends have shown me, incontestably, that life is about more than just eating or drinking whatever you want, whenever you want it.

On the other hand, if a person isn't ill, why deny oneself pleasurable experiences for the sake of living to be 90 or 100? And what would be the good of living to be that old if there's no one left to party with? We know that restraint in matters of food and drink, combined with devotion to exercise and stress management, do not win a person immortality.

HELP IS AT HAND

I offer this book to help you figure out a winning health strategy. When do you take that "extra card," and when do you pass on it? What can you do to compensate for those times when you take one card or more too many? Thus *The Healthy Hedonist* will assist you in finding a balance between having fun on weekends and holidays with friends and family and managing to stay on top of the weekday grind—whatever it is that creates cash flow to pay the bills. Though my approach is scientifically and philosophically based (see Chapter 4), I'm presenting suggestions in an easy-to-follow sequence—showing how you could implement them, starting from when you wake on a weekday morning until it's time to go to sleep at night. I describe how the concept works with several kinds of weekends—the busy ones, the socially indulgent ones and the relaxing, restorative ones.

This book is not about the obvious. Nowhere in it will I tell you that smoking is dangerous to your health. I assume you know that. I won't tell you to lose weight. If you're overweight, I assume you've tried. There are lots of other books out there addressing those issues.

Since working moms are among the busiest people on the planet, my suggestions are often aimed at their schedule demands. But if you are not a working mom, be assured that I'm not just thinking of moms as I write. My hunch is that if the suggestions work for moms, they will probably work for dads, singles or couples without children. I've tried to make my book as inclusive as possible. I ask you to forgive references or suggestions that may not be specific to you.

Very importantly, if the suggestions in my book sound simple, it's because they are. But they have great power when you implement them with consistency. Small things done with regularity can have a wondrous effect. This doesn't have to be hard!

And finally, dear reader, as many suggestions as I've managed to include, I don't think for a split second that I've figured out all the angles to healthy hedonism. I invite you to share your experiences and ideas at *thehealthyhedonist.com*. I hope that as we share ideas on how to make healthy hedonism work, we will all find new ways to be healthier while enjoying life to the max! What a wonderful quest!

"We'll never know the worth of water till the well go dry."

18th-century Scottish proverb

"Ask yourself if your job, your family or your recreational habits are causing you to become a 'dry well.' Is your lifestyle 'sustainable'?"

Chapter Two

THE DRY WELL

"Burn-out" describes the situation that occurs when an individual becomes overloaded with responsibilities and can no longer function at a high level of performance. Unless reversed, burn-out may lead to depression or chronic illness.

THE ISSUE OF SUSTAINABLILITY

Before describing how healthy hedonism can help prevent burn-out, I'd like to introduce a word here that's often used in environmental literature, but rarely applied to personal lifestyle. The word is *"sustainability."* With regard to the environment, it refers to whether a human activity will damage an ecosystem's ability to maintain itself.

An aquifer is a simple example. Aquifers are underground water sources created by rainwater that has percolated down past rock and soil over thousands of years to fill deep areas of sand or gravel. We tap into these aquifers for use in farming, for personal use and for manufacturing purposes. But we have tended to take the water out more rapidly than it is replenished by natural processes. So there may come a point when a particular aquifer will pump dry. Agriculture and other human uses that depend on such an aquifer can be called "unsustainable."

Similarly, ask yourself if your job, your family or your recreational habits are causing you to become a "dry well." Is your lifestyle "sustainable"? Will your current diet and physical activities allow you to maintain your health and sense of fun well past the age of retirement? If you can truthfully answer "yes," then you have already achieved balance in your life. But if you answer "no," consider what you might do about it.

HOW TO WORK WITH THIS BOOK

The purpose of this book is not to give you all the answers. You will have to think through your unique situation and make some difficult choices on your own. However, *The Healthy Hedonist* can guide you on the path of physical, mental and emotional self-care, and as a result, you'll find more energy and resilience with which to maintain and improve your life. By beginning with these small changes, you can establish a physical and psychological beachhead from which to launch bigger changes.

What those changes will be depends on your situation. Perhaps your current goal is to continue to grow in your professional career, taking on higher and higher levels of responsibility. Perhaps it's to switch your career to one that is more in line with your philosophies or less personally exploitive. Perhaps it's to go back to school. Maybe it's to get out of a toxic relationship or to tackle an addiction. It could be to just keep yourself together long enough to get your kids out of school and on their own. Or it might be to fulfill your obligation to your parents by looking after them in their old age. The demands of your life will determine how much you need to counterbalance the stress with healthy and restorative practices.

Much of the information in this book is very basic. Perhaps you're already familiar with much of it. If so, that's great! With the healthy pleasurable activities you've already incorporated, give yourself the opportunity to enjoy them more deeply. Try to appreciate each occasion as though you'd never experienced anything like it before. Or if many of the ideas are new to you, try them out with a sense of adventure. As you progress, you'll find that the benefits you gain are worth a little effort and that this process can be fun!

In our own lives, each of us is the goose that lays the golden eggs. The ability to meet the needs of others flows from the ability to meet our own needs. You probably already know this on some level and you may be thinking that the realization that you need to care for yourself doesn't put extra hours in the day. It doesn't take away responsibilities. It doesn't give you extra cash. So how does one accomplish this self-nurturing and self-care without taking away time and resources legitimately owed to work and family? You're about to find out.

HAVE DOUBTS?

Just in case you have some little nagging doubts as to whether you can justify flinging yourself headlong into healthy hedonism—in case you have some notion that this form of hedonism might be selfish—the answer is a resounding "NO," and here's why:

In this crazy world, we're *all* experiencing lots of stress, and I don't have to create a litany of all the sources.

Melanie Beattie, author of *Codependent No More*, states that while it is normal to *react* to stress, it is also heroic and lifesaving to learn how to not simply react, but instead act in more healthy ways. And she admits that most of us need help to learn how to do that.

Just let me repeat the essence of this. Instead of reacting to stress, we need to act in healthy ways, and this can be heroic and lifesaving. (Whose life will you be saving? Your own!)

Try out the ideas in this book with an open mind as to how they can work for you. Some may work "as is." Others may need a nip and tuck to fit smoothly into your busy lifestyle. As you consider these adjustments, don't try to make too many all at once. As my dad used to say, with a big grin on his face, "Keep the picture on the tube. Just turn one knob at a time!"

"All we need is to uncover the subset of activities that are both healthy and intrinsically pleasurable."

Chapter Three

THE LOST KEY

A PHILOSOPHICAL FOUNDATION

Probably everyone has had the experience of searching high and low for a set of keys. Someone else comes in the room and says, "Oh yeah. They're right over there." Our sense of relief from finding the keys is mixed with some exasperation that it took so long and caused so much confusion.

The search for a set of keys is going on in the world of preventive healthcare information. The folks in charge just haven't been looking in the right place.

In *Pleasures and Pains: A Theory of Qualitative Hedonism*, Rem B. Edwards, a professor of philosophy at the University of Tennessee, inadvertently discovered the flaw in most current preventive health information. Dr. Edwards asserts, "Long-run hedonism does not say that we should act to maximize merely *future* pleasures, but pleasures over the whole span of life, which *includes the present and immediate future* as well as the distant future."

Why is it impossible to talk about "future" pleasures? Because, as Dr. Edwards reminds us, "In a sense, the future never comes; and any philosophy that advocates the actualization of merely distant future pleasures requires a continual postponement of enjoyment for the sake of that future which never comes." He therefore takes a solid philosophical stand, affirming that long-run hedonism includes, rather than excludes, enjoyment in the present and immediate future, "since its ideal is that of happiness over the *entire* span of life."

Many philosophies and even pure semantics tell us that the future never arrives. By definition of the word, if the future arrived into the now, it would no longer be the future. We have only The Now. Consequently, any healthcare regime that asks us to engage in painful, unpleasant or just bland and boring behavior in the present for the sake of health in the "future" is sort of like buying questionable real estate. Sure, it could appreciate, but in the meantime, do you want to live in that neighborhood?

This is more than philosophical debate. In this century, the major threats to long-term health have become heart disease, diabetes and cancer, all of which are known to have major lifestyle components to their causes. Despite widespread public education stretching over decades, the rates of obesity and diabetes are skyrocketing. Heart disease remains a leading cause of death, and cancer is not far behind. *Obviously, a lot of people are not able to apply the widely available health information to their lives.*

But wait! Maybe there's something wrong with the information. Or could it be that healthcare educators and practitioners haven't presented all the options to the "short-term" hedonists? Maybe they haven't dissected this issue sufficiently to discover what is both healthy and pleasurable, with the emphasis on the latter, thank you.

REWARDS VS. PUNISHMENT

If you studied Psychology 101, you may remember how lab rats could always be trained toward certain behaviors with rewards and away from other behaviors with punishment. The experiments demonstrated the reward and punishment circuit in the brain and were the basic psychological premise of the psychological school called *"behaviorism."* I never thought behaviorism could adequately explain all human motivations, but it certainly explains why a lot of exercise programs don't work!

Let's use the example of golf. For all of you who love golf, I'm not trying to talk you out of your enjoyment of the game. I just want to let you know that it wasn't fun for me. I spent an entire college semester at the driving range, trying to learn to hit the golf ball. Then I actually tried to play nine holes with my mother, a reasonably good player. Unfortunately for my future as a golfer, I committed the cardinal sin of holding up the foursome behind us. I hit the ball first into one rough, and then into the opposite one, with subsequent delays in the ball discovery process. I haven't forgotten my embarrassment. It was anything but fun. Could I have learned to play golf competently if I'd stuck with it? Undoubtedly. I just wasn't willing to chance a repeat of the discomfort I'd experienced.

At approximately the same time, I learned to ski. After only one day, I reached a point of exhilaration in skiing that made it gratifying beyond words. It later became an activity that had spiritual overtones, giving me a sense of freedom and a feeling of union with the natural world.

The difference between the two experiences shows how I came to understand why many people have trouble finding a form of exercise that provides enough immediate gratification to help them past initial feelings of bumbling incompetence, humiliation and physical discomfort. Most sports have social components. If we could learn them without anyone ever seeing us until we were good at them, there might be more people involved. Rollerblading is another example of that for me. It's something I think I might like to learn, but my personal need is to be able to learn it in an empty roller rink, not down on Southern California's famous Venice Beach with hundreds of groovy people watching. My dignity is far more fragile than my physical body.

In a somewhat similar way, a lot of healthy food involves a learning curve. For those whose taste buds are programmed to other tastes, the idea of eating five servings of fruits and vegetables a day may seem like a prison sentence in a rabbit hutch. That's because many people have never received pleasure and gratification from eating salads, stir fries and steamed veggies. To seek pleasure and gratification from food is basic. If the healthcare community says, "Eat five to seven servings of fruits and vegetables a day" without providing a direct experience of how pleasurable that can be, it's little wonder that too few people follow the guidelines.

But frankly, this doesn't have to be difficult. All we need to do is uncover the subset of activities that are both healthy and intrinsically pleasurable. The chart on the following pages presents a glance at many of these. It provides a visual way to begin to understand how the Five Pillars of Healthy Hedonism work together. In the chapter that follows, I'll explain in greater detail.

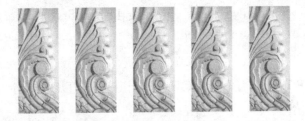

FIVE PILLARS OF HEALTHY HEDONISM

Here's where the fun comes in! Look at the Pillars Chart. It shows how the activities of healthy hedonism fall into five general categories. Many of the activities offer the promise of pure hedonistic pleasure, with no apologies whatsoever. Now pick the easiest, most inviting activity from one of the columns. It could be something you're already doing.

When you've started enjoying the benefits of that activity, congratulate yourself. Engage in it more passionately!

THE FIVE PILLARS OF HEALTHY HEDONISM

Positive Stimulation	Stress Reduction	Quality of Food
Love	Gently Waking *chapter 5*	Lots of Fruit *chapter 6*
Spiritual Connectedness	*Deep Breathing* *chapter 11*	Protein in a.m., Carbohydrates at Night, *chapter 9*
Whatever You Enjoy Doing	Music, Flowers & Candles, *chapter 14*	Soy, *chapter 9*
Special Occasions, Being with those you enjoy *chapters 18–23*	Aromatherapy *chapter 15*	The Right Kinds of Fats, *chapter 13*
Anticipation, Planning something pleasurable	Bathing, *chapter 16*	Snacks, *chapter 13*
	Prayer, Meditation & Journal Writing, *chapter 17*	Juicing & Saturday Salads *chapter 20*
Hobbies	Better Sleep *chapter 18*	Cooking with Friends *chapter 21*
Goals & Optimism (Conclusion)	Yoga, *chapter 26*	Eating Out & Travel, *chapter 22*
	Spa Experience *chapter 28*	

Now add an activity from one of the other columns. Embrace and enjoy it, too! When you've embarked on an activity from each of the five pillars, you will begin to feel the intensified effect of the healthy hedonist lifestyle. You could stop there, but you'll feel even better if you add a second activity from each column, then a third, and so on. Chapter 4 explains each of these categories and how they work together to help you feel more alive and energetic, in effect, a *totally* healthy hedonist.

Circulation	Detox for Health	
Exercise, all forms but esp. Walking *chapter 7*	Fruits, *chapter 6*	
	Detox Bathing *chapter 16*	
Dry Skin Brushing *chapter 8*	Vitamins & Minerial *chapter 17*	
Dancing *chapter 22*	Juicing, *chapter 20*	*Healthy Hedonism is not just about food, relaxation techniques, or exercise. It's about all of these and more....*
Yoga & T'ai Chi *chapter 26*	Detox Teas *chapter 23*	
Massage *chapter 27*	Weekend Detox *chapter 25*	
Saunas *chapter 28*	Pure Drinking Water, *chapter 25*	
	Saunas, *chapter 28*	

"Happiness is critical to health. This seems like a no-brainer until we find ourselves mired in work commitments or problem relationships."

Chapter Four

PILLARS OF HEALTHY HEDONISM

There are five pillars of scientific research that support the premise of healthy hedonism.

Each of these areas has been covered in great detail in hundreds of books and magazines by persons with excellent credentials. Several are referenced in the Notes and Resources sections for various chapters. My purpose in this chapter is to reassure you that the health benefits the different pillars provide have been documented through rigorous, well-established scientific research.

What's different here is the way of looking at how the parts contribute to the whole. In terms of functionality, the elements work very much like major parts of a car. Surprisingly so.

Positive stimulation functions much like the gas pedal of a car. We all enjoy that surge of power in a well-engineered automobile. Major aspects of our life—such as love, faith, goals, ambitions, anticipation of all kinds, and doing whatever you enjoy—provide the motivation that gets you out of bed in the morning and through the day. You may take theses sources of motivation for granted, unless you don't have them. My point is that you need to cultivate different types of positive stimulation in your life.

Stress reduction acts like the brakes of a car. No one wants to be in a moving car that has no brakes. Similarly, if you have no way to control the pace of your life, it's easy to find yourself wrecked, in a figurative sense. You need to be able to slow things down, such as your heart rate and your adrenal glands. The great news is that there are many hedonistic pleasures that can help you do that.

Quality of food compares to the quality of fuel that you use in your car. You know your car will run better if you offer it something more than inferior fuel. Your body is the same way. With the human body, the timing of when you eat certain substances also has a lot to do with how well you feel.

Circulation in the body can be compared to the action of a car's fuel and oil pumps. Both a car and the human body do better when they're regularly moving, not sitting. You've experienced how a car that's not been driven regularly sputters and coughs until all the fluids have been circulated and all the parts have been relubricated. In the same way, if you don't move all your body parts regularly, you're going to feel stiff and sluggish.

Detox is like changing the oil filter in your car periodically. It's wise to replace the filter from time to time so it can remove impurities from the oil that would otherwise clog up the system. With your body, the direct equivalent of taking out the oil filter and putting in a new one would be a liver transplant, which is not your best option! Detox is something that you can do on an ongoing basis through your choices in food and drink, as well as with supplements and activities such as saunas and detox bathing. But it can also be accomplished in discrete intervals such as detox weekends.

That's a quick look at how the five pillars work together to improve the functionality of your body. The payoff is in terms of energy and mood. Once everything's working better, you're going to feel better and life will be more fun. More fun begets more fun.

The rest of this book presents the activities, based on these five pillars, that you can use to achieve your own version of healthy hedonism. Many of these behaviors, techniques or strategies may be things you're familiar with or that you already do to some extent. Those are the ones that should attract special attention. If they're already a part of your life, adjusting them is easier than creating a new habit, which takes a lot more energy. This book may suggest ways to draw greater pleasure and benefit from things you're already doing.

Back to the First Pillar.

POSITIVE STIMULATION

Enjoyment is a nicer word for positive stimulation, with its root in the word "joy." However, joy does not communicate the breadth of experience that falls under this category. The first pillar includes knowing that you are loved and accepted, that you have bonds to close friends and family. It includes spiritual connectedness, a deeply held belief that your consciousness continues past death, and that, ultimately, all shall be well.

This category varies widely because what each of us considers fun varies. I love to spend time with friends and family. Some people don't.

Conversely, gardening—my husband's passion—is okay as far as I'm concerned, but I don't derive a sense of anticipation from it. On the other hand, I might look forward for months to an upcoming ballet performance.

Much of the benefit from this category may come from the planning of activities. Anticipation has a tremendously positive effect on personal health. Planning a vacation, for example, can, in some ways, be more fun than the vacation itself. You experience the pure joy of possibilities in the planning stage—no luggage hassles, no screwed-up reservations. There's that great buildup of excitement as the day of departure comes closer and closer. And finally, hallelujah! The day arrives and you're ready to go. That feeling is so important that I strongly recommend that everybody should always be planning something! It doesn't have to be expensive. It could be a camping trip, a picnic, or the cheapest seats to a performance, but the point is to make your plans special and enjoy them during the weeks and months while you're planning.

The scientific research that validates positive stimulation is varied.

Early psychological research showed that baby monkeys suffered tremendous psychological damage if they didn't have a "mommy" to cling to. It showed that physical touch and the sense of care it communicates play important parts in the development of our nervous systems. Without it, we fail to thrive.

Research further shows that emotional health is a major determinant for how long a person will live—happy people live longer than unhappy ones, based on ratings of their emotional stability.

Then there's *"psychoneuroimmunology."* It's a long word for a new field of research showing that our mental state and immune systems are linked. It explains why you're more likely to get sick when you're under a lot of stress; the stress wears down your immune system and leaves you a sitting duck for a bug. Conversely, when you're happy, your immune system is stronger. The classic example of this is the story of how Norman Cousins used laughter as an essential element to reverse a crippling disease, which he documented in his book, *Anatomy of an Illness*.

Not the least of these areas is spiritual support, which gives us the ability to endure hard times. Research has shown that persons with religious beliefs live longer than those without them.

The point is that happiness is critical to health. This seems like a "no-brainer," but the issue becomes more complex when we find ourselves mired in personal and work commitments or problem relationships. Nonetheless, one can't indefinitely ignore either unhappiness or the feeling of being overwhelmed. The First Pillar serves as a reminder that there comes a point where, for the sake of our physical health, we need to deal with the emotional issues that may be making us unhappy. If this reminds you of your situation, do you have someone in your life who gives you shelter, who can help you sort it out? If you don't, find someone. If you need to, pay someone.

This pillar is also about making time for close friends, family and the things you enjoy. If your schedule makes that difficult, find a way to simplify your life. A statement frequently repeated is that no one wishes on their deathbed that they'd spent more time at the office.

STRESS REDUCTION
The Second Pillar is stress reduction or relaxation. There's been a lot of research to prove how damaging stress can be. Most people are aware of that. A challenge of mod-

ern life is to find relaxation techniques that fit with modern lifestyles.

Our bodies have changed very little in the time since the last Ice Age. We are not so physically different from our ancestors. The "flight or fight" response gave them the ability to outmaneuver a tiger, or to bring down a wooly mammoth. The same physical response mechanism still operates for us. A surge of adrenaline is released when we're in a stressful situation, but the difference is that we're not out on the high plains running off the powerful stress hormones. Instead, we're sitting in traffic, breathing smog, and trying to suppress our emotions, day after day.

In the good news column, there are lots of ways to reduce stress. Some of them, such as yoga, meditation and deep breathing, you've heard about dozens of times. These are like investment "banks." The more you bring, the more you'll take away. The benefits they provide will increase dramatically as you become more aware and are able to better focus on them. They have the potential to transform your life.

In terms of hedonistic pleasures, this category also includes activities that feel totally indulgent, such as aromatherapy, bathing and the whole spa experience. Knowing how important these activities can be to your health should help you to schedule and justify them, because there's no doubt that you will enjoy yourself once you've begun experimenting with them.

This category is so rich that I ran out of room to list everything on the chart that could be included; for example, massage and saunas qualify under stress relief.

QUALITY OF FOOD

There's no way to summarize 30 years of research into nutrition in a couple of paragraphs. Clearly and indisputably, the Third Pillar, food, has an effect on our health. Most of us know that. What has been harder is figuring *how* to do what we know is good for us.

My tips on this huge subject are scattered throughout the book. More specifically, Chapter 9, "Rediscovering Energy," describes new findings that can have a tremendous difference in how you feel. I'm happy to report that it has more to do with *when* you eat certain foods than with what you eat, and this knowledge can give you a more flexible framework for adjusting your diet.

Chapter 13, "Tasty Right-Fat Snacks," offers the combined wisdom of my most attractive friends on ways to nibble without having any reason to feel guilty later.

CIRCULATION

The Fourth Pillar is circulation, and I use the word to refer to those activities that improve the ability of your blood and lymphatic fluid to circulate. The effect is to bring more oxygen to every cell of the body and carry away toxins to the bowels, kidneys and skin for excretion. This has the effect of giving you more energy.

There's no doubt that regular exercise is the most effective way to do this. The health benefits of exercise in terms of lowering the risk of heart disease, diabetes and numerous other serious chronic diseases are well known. But this book does not spend a lot of time on this particular subject area because it is so widely covered elsewhere. This does not mean that it's unimportant. Whatever form of exercise anyone can integrate is great. I'm a real cheerleader for walking, as I find it requires the least organizational effort—just walking shoes. Also, you don't have to spend too much time at it to achieve results—15 to 30 minutes a day. Besides, it's very pleasurable.

There are a few other physical activities that qualify as pretty darn easy to manage. You'll find them in Chapter 7, "Walk, Walk, Walk—Around the Block."

I never mean to be a nag, though, so if you're not yet into a habit of exercise, you can ease into it while using other means to increase your circulation. These include massage. I don't think I need to tell you how pleasurable massage is, so if you can afford it, call soon for an appointment.

For those who can't afford regular massage, this book offers a few other techniques that anyone can afford. They include dry skin brushing and saunas. These activities are stimulating in themselves, and they just feel good.

DETOXIFICATION

The Fifth Pillar, detoxification, is an extremely important aspect of life in our post-modern world. Most of us are exposed to hundreds of chemicals every day. That, combined with poor choices in diet, lack of exercise, and not enough water or nutrients, causes our livers to become backlogged with its detox duties. The result is fatigue, depression, lethargy, poor complexion, bad breath and an array of possible illnesses, cancer being the scariest of them all.

The strategies in this book that come under the "Detox for Health" pillar are everyday activities such as eating and juicing fruits and vegetables, taking the right combination of antioxidant vitamins and minerals, and drinking filtered water and "detox" herbal teas. Several "spa" activities including detox bathing and saunas, also promote the body's natural detoxification capabilities, and these can be as luxurious as they are beneficial.

Chapter 25 is entirely devoted to the subject of detox and suggests a "Detox Weekend" approach. It will give you an overview of how the body's organs and systems work together to eliminate toxins, a function that's essential to good health. An understanding of detox can become a powerful tool in your efforts to protect and enhance the quality of your life.

Now that you have some understanding of how the Pillars of Healthy Hedonism work together, I'll explain how elements from all the pillars can fit easily and naturally into the course of your weekdays and weekends.

Part Two

Week-long Pleasures

"How we start the day is important. All of us deserve the luxury of coming out of our sleep state gently, even if we can't doze as long as we wish."

Chapter Five

Wake Me Gently, Please

There you are, happily snoozing away, enjoying a great dream. And all of a sudden, that sweet reverie is interrupted by a terrible noise.

How we start the day is important. All of us deserve the luxury of coming out of our sleep state gently, even if we can't doze as long as we wish.

I have a friend who says that the name "alarm" clock ought to tell you right away that it's a bad way to wake up. Who wants to awaken to adrenaline overload, the very first thing in the morning? Wouldn't it make sense to save that response for a real emergency?

Here's the good news. Several developments in the world of clocks now offer more gentle ways to wake up each morning.

THE ZEN CLOCK

The first new option is called the Zen Clock (see Resources in the back of this book to learn where to find one). Having tried it, I'm happy to report that this is a most peaceful alternative to the jarring and heart-stopping alarm clock that arouses most people every day.

The first wake-up chime is soft and you might miss it. The chime vibrates for about a minute. A long pause follows, minutes long, before the next chime, which is slightly more insistent. This one might start to reach your consciousness. More chimes follow, each a bit stronger and closer in time to the next. Finally, you have to admit it's time to get up. But you could certainly lie in bed and listen to the chimes and be quite content.

A sleeping spouse doesn't even stir, as long as you don't abuse the privilege and let the chimes keep chiming—and chiming—and chiming....

For those interested in remembering and keeping track of dreams, the clock slows the transition from sleeping to waking. This makes it much easier to retain the memory of a dream long enough to write it down.

The Zen Clock can also be very helpful in a yoga or meditation practice, where you would hardly wish to use an alarm clock to end your sessions. It's even proven to be beneficial in meetings as a gentle way to remind speakers to "wind it up."

Though sophisticated in terms of its tonal qualities, the Zen Clock is simple enough for anyone to use. It's housed in a lovely triangular wooden body and comes in a number of styles, including a travel version.

OTHER ALTERNATIVES

A new, more sophisticated breed of clock radio offers many of the same benefits as the Zen Clock through different capabilities. Included are a CD player, a radio and a "nature sounds" sleep feature. Though more complex to use than the Zen Clock, it's a pleasant technological challenge. Imagine falling asleep every night to the sound of waves, wind, rain or a forest. Imagine waking up to the gradually increasing volume of your favorite mellow morning music. Two manufacturers have similar versions of this clock. (See Resources.) One is more expensive than the other, but both are great deals in terms of what they can do for your mornings.

Still another kind of clock offers a gradually brightening light that wakens you gently, like a real sunrise. It begins with a faint glow, gradually becoming brighter until you are eased awake in a pleasantly lit room. This clock can also do the opposite, giving you a way to fall asleep while reading, without having to turn off the light. (Again, consult the Resources section.)

WORTH THE PRICE

Healthy hedonism is more a matter of attitude than money. As you read the rest of the book, you'll see the emphasis is on solutions that require very little, if any, outlay of cash.

But if you can't just sleep until you naturally wake up, my best suggestion for improving the way your day begins is to invest in one of these clocks. Each of them makes it possible for you to gently make the transition from sleeping to waking, from dreaming to smiling, instead of being jerked into the work-a-day world time after time.

The cost of the clocks described above ranges from $99 to $220. All of them are well worth the cost for anyone willing to pay a few cents a day to wake up more pleasantly for years to come. All carry money-back guarantees and one-year warranties. Think what such a clock could do for your mood each morning, and consequently for your whole household as well as for the guy who cuts you off on the freeway and the associate who dumps a new load of work in your in-basket as soon as you sit down at your desk.

If you can't afford one of these immediately, print out the pages from the websites mentioned in Resources, drop some hints around the time of your birthday or the winter holidays, or sell a few household items you're not using and apply the proceeds to the purchase of the clock. This is something you will use and it will make a difference in the way you feel from Day One.

These are also wonderful gift ideas for someone who has to wake up early.

Now that you're blissfully awake, the day's first adventure awaits.

"Does your mouth water at the suggestion of a big, ripe, juicy summer peach, with a smell that brings to mind hot summer afternoons?"

Chapter Six

FRUIT, NATURE'S FAST FOOD

One of the reasons I'm healthy is that I eat a lot of fruit. As a hedonist, I only eat the ones I like, which happens to be almost all of them. Of course, all hedonists love food, all kinds of food, for all kinds of reasons. The equation—food equals pleasure—is an easy one. It made sense to us even when we were babies.

What's different about a healthy hedonist's approach to food? The healthy hedonist appreciates not just the sight, smell, texture and taste of food, but the effect it has on the body—both short and long term. Taste may still be the number one consideration, but it has to be placed in balance with a food's nutritional considerations.

As a healthy hedonist, I'm not trying to persuade you to eat something you're sure you'll never like—the way mothers try to talk their children into developing a taste for spinach. Rather, my goal is to increase your appreciation for something I feel confident you already enjoy and to suggest ways to not only derive more pleasure from that food, but to eat more of it.

Let's first consider fruit for its sensual nature, beauty, smell, taste and how these qualities affect our imagination. Then we'll consider its convenience and, finally, the health benefits. On all of these, fruit scores high.

THE WONDERS OF FRUIT

There's no more beautiful food than fruit. We first eat it with our eyes. In terms of looks, fruit is an easy "10." There are scientific explanations for the color of fruit. It comes from plant components called phytonutrients. Color is important because it attract birds. They spread the seed, allowing the plant to propagate itself to areas further than the reach of the tree's branches. The phytonutrients also protect the fruit and its seeds from overexposure to the sun while the fruit is maturing.

Did you ever notice that a lot of fruit comes in the same colors as the sunset? Maybe it's because fruit literally embodies the sun. Fruit must have inspired Renaissance artists. Those warm Florentine colors—deep to light reds, oranges, pale yellows to mellow golds, and purples—are all tones found in the fruit that grows so well in a Mediterranean climate.

As beautiful as flowers on your kitchen table, fruit makes a wonderful edible centerpiece. When you stop to think about what's happening, watching fruit is awe-inspiring. Fruit is alive. There are enzymes at work within, bringing the fruit to its peak of ripeness, and then beyond.

MAKING YOUR SELECTIONS

Our marvelous food distribution system brings us fruit from all over the world throughout the year. The very essence of the calendar—the fruits of the season, the passing of the year—is embodied and experienced in each piece of fruit.

While the quality of our food supply has deteriorated

in many ways—due to over-processing, additives, etc.—the availability of fruit is something to cheer about. The variety of fruit in the average supermarket today is something even the wealthiest people never had in the past.

Many hands, much knowledge and a great deal of infrastructure are invested in every piece of fruit you see at a grocery store. Give a thought to the farm workers, packers, truckers and grocers who bring you a treat worthy of a king. Fruit isn't manufactured in a giant factory. It has to be very carefully handled each step of the way as it speeds to market.

Organic fruit is best for you, and if you have access and can afford this, it is well worth it. But well-washed conventionally grown fresh fruit is also incomparably better for you than its canned equivalents.

Let's consider our possible fruit choices...

Apples are great year-round, but unparalleled in autumn. The selection now available ranges from tart to sweet, green to yellow to red, with shades in between. There's even a new variety called "Pink Ladies." Highly sensual *pomegranates* and *persimmons* also become available in the fall.

Tangerines remind me of Christmas when my mother put them in our stockings.

Grapefruit and *oranges* bring sunshine to mid-winter.

Strawberries mean spring.

In the middle of summer, the most sensual fruits—stone fruits—become ripe. The stone fruits include *peaches, plums, cherries* and *apricots. Grapes,* in a hedonistic class by themselves with their connotations of wine and revelry, also become abundant in mid-summer. There are also all the wonderful varieties of *melons,* so cool and clean-tasting.

Does your mouth water at the suggestion of a big, ripe,

juicy summer peach, with a smell that brings to mind hot summer afternoons, picnics and swimming pools? Should we not also mention how fruit can recreate for us the memories of when you actually could take the summer off?

What memories do *watermelons* bring to your mind? Remember getting so sticky eating your fill of watermelon that the only real answer was to rinse off under the garden hose. Was that fun or what? Maybe we should try that again!

What would it be worth to you to be able to bring some of the joys of childhood back to your morning and afternoon snacks? With a little effort, you can become a true adventurer in search of the best fruit in your neighborhood, hunting it down for the romance and beauty it can bring to your day. Which store within your weekly driving rounds has the best? Is it a farmer's market on the weekends, or a little out-of-the-way ethnic grocery? Maybe it's a gourmet grocer. If you have questions about how to choose a fruit or how to tell if it's ripe, ask the produce manager. If you bring the manager into your sense of adventure, you'll do something positive for both of you. Also, try making a point of stopping at produce stands when you travel past them.

And the reward for these adventures? Once a year, for each kind of fruit, you'll find one that offers an explosion of taste. When you find that "best of season" piece of fruit, it tells you, in a bite, that life is still very much to be savored. I had that experience recently. It was a yellow "Manila Mango," just a little more tart than the other varieties, but what a difference that made! I went back to the store and bought six more.

All sorts of exotic fruit species appear in the stores during the course of the year. Have you ever had an *elephant heart plum*? Watch for them in late summer. And *blood or-*

anges. It used to be that they only grew in Spain. What a surprise of color waits for you inside!

And there are exotic tropical fruits to be experienced, including *guava, passion fruit* and, if you're very lucky, *cherimoya.* If you have an encyclopedia handy, or even a dictionary with a lot of pictures, you can increase your appreciation of the fruit experience by looking up such new choices. The other day, I asked my husband, who traveled for years in the tropics, about *papayas.* To me, they seemed too big to grow on a tree. However, since they're not melons, I knew they must grow on trees. Patrick says the tree is rather small, only about 10 feet tall. The fruit grows close to the main trunk and each tree bears a small number of fruit. Knowing this increased my appreciation for papaya because I knew there were only a few from each tree.

Mangoes, on the other hand, come from very large trees, bearing loads of fruit. Knowing that makes me want to eat more mangoes. Mango mania stretches from late spring into the middle of summer.

Next time you go to the market, just take a moment to stop in the produce section and first enjoy the spectrum of colors. Then close your eyes for a moment and smell. What individual fruits does your nose detect? Then start snooping around a bit and try something—at least one fruit— that you haven't had for a long time, or ever.

You've probably heard that five to seven servings of fruits and vegetables per day are recommended. But if you are not in the habit of eating numerous pieces of fresh fruit each day, here are a few more tips on how to fit them in.

DON'T OVERLOOK SMOOTHIES
Smoothies are a great way to get a couple of pieces of

fruit down in a hurry. If you combine them with protein powder and a tablespoon or two of flaxseed oil (an Omega 3 oil with tremendous health benefits, explained more fully in Chapter 13), you will have gone a long way in a couple of minutes toward your daily nutritional requirements. And you can make that smoothie portable—carry it around the house while you're getting ready to go to work, or take it with you in the car.

A blender that has a screw-off blade assembly is much easier to wash. Rinse the pitcher part out immediately after making the smoothie and then just give the insides, including the blades, a quick sweep with a bottle brush so the protein powder doesn't harden. That way, cleaning the blender won't be a formidable chore later for either you or the dishwasher.

Smoothies are a great way to use fruit that's just a tad too ripe to enjoy all by itself. Very ripe fruit blends much more easily and tastes great. Smoothies are also a good way to use fruit that isn't quite as flavorful as you'd hoped it would be. An unexceptional peach, for example, gives a nice flavor to a smoothie, even if it would be disappointing on its own.

THE FRUIT CONVENIENCE FACTOR

Fresh fruit is the original "fast food." It requires no preparation other than washing.

A positive aspect about indulging yourself in one or two pieces of fruit, first thing in the morning, is that you've then made a significant dent in your daily fruit and vegetable requirement, with very little effort in terms of preparation.

Bananas are credited as being "America's favorite fruit," and we go through a lot of them in our house too. They have many great qualities, but they're not as great as apples for carrying around—too easily bruised. So, for us, bananas tend to be an "at home" fruit.

Here are two reasons why I've voted *apples* as my all-time "best friend" fruit.

1. It has been said that evolution designed our hands for picking and eating fruit. Watching a chimp eat a banana demonstrates this. A whole medium-sized apple fits so easily in the space between your thumb and middle finger, it's almost uncanny. This makes apples very neat and easy to eat in your car.

2. Apples are rarely so juicy as to be messy. If you find one that is, it's probably a great-tasting fresh autumn apple, and you're going to forgive the messiness. Just close your eyes and think of how wonderful autumn and apples are (but not if you're driving!). During the rest of the year, though tasty and crisp, apples are a neat treat, and that means you can eat them while wearing good clothes on the way to or from work and meetings.

Here are some ideas for working apples into your life at other times than just first thing in the morning.

On the weekend, when you go to the market, buy some beautiful apples. As soon as you arrive home, dump them in a basin in the sink, and wash and polish the apples with a clean kitchen towel. Then arrange them in a nice bowl situated in a highly visible spot. Alternatively, you could wrap the apples individually in paper towels and then in sandwich bags, or secure the wrapping with a rubber band. Voila! They're now a healthy, convenient on-the-go food that you can throw in your purse, briefcase, backpack or lunch box. Last, but not least, remember that apples are wonderfully filling, especially considering how low they are in calories. A medium-sized apple has about 80 calories, no fat, and lots of fiber.

Oranges come a close second in my fruit popularity contest, again because they're so dependable. I like peeling them, ripping back the rind with my hands so that citrus oil squirts into the room and fills it with the smell of orange.

HOW & WHEN TO EAT FRUIT

First thing in the morning is one of the best times of the day to eat fruit. It can pass through your stomach within a half hour as long as you eat the fruit all by itself. That's part of its healthiness.

To improve digestion, the recommendation is that fruit, which is high in natural sugar, is best eaten alone. This means it is better not to eat it with or after other foods. This is more true of some fruits than others. For example, if you've ever experienced indigestion from melon, try eating some separately from other foods. From this perspective, fruit doesn't make either a good salad or dessert item. Fruit is especially good either first thing in the morning or when the stomach has had time to empty, say in the middle of the morning or afternoon. Fruits digest rapidly, so other foods can be eaten within a half-hour or so. For that reason, fruit can make a great choice to stave off hunger in the hour or two before dinner. This is a great time to eat apples. Since the fruit has no fat and is low in calories, it won't ruin a diet. Actually, apple slices make very nice "chips." They're crisp but don't break apart, and you can dip them in any number of flavorful concoctions. (See Chapter 13, "Tasty, Right-Fat Snacks.")

One of the hardest parts of enjoying fruit at their finest

may be to develop the patience to wait until they reach the peak of perfection. But if you do, it's worth the wait. There's no food so elegant as a perfectly ripe *pear*. Most fruit doesn't have nearly as much flavor if eaten before its time. In addition, fruit doesn't have as much flavor cold. If you can eat your supply before it over-ripens at room temperature, I think it's best to leave the fruit out once you bring it home, meanwhile enjoying the beauty. If you prefer to refrigerate it, consider bringing the fruit out the night before so it has plenty of time to reach room temperature before morning.

Interestingly enough, the nutritional value of most fruits increases up to the point of being fully ripe. This is also true of *berries* and *cherries*.

THE HEALTH BENEFITS OF FRUIT

An apple a day keeps the doctor away. It's funny how accurate that old expression is. Decades later, we find that all the literature on detoxification and immune support, not to mention cancer and heart disease prevention, stresses how important fresh fruits and vegetables are to health.

It has become widespread knowledge that fruits and vegetables have significant cancer-preventing qualities. We're going to skip an extended explanation of why, because this information is available from a lot of other sources. (See Notes.) Notice how your mouth feels after you swallow a piece of fruit. It feels clean. Fruit, when eaten alone, helps clean your entire digestive system, beginning with your teeth and gums. Fruit provides lots of water and fiber to keep you regular. And what a nice way to facilitate that essential process.

Fruit is also wonderfully detoxifying. A short fruit fast, explained in Chapter 25, "Detox Weekends," is a great way to begin experimenting with personal detoxification techniques.

Fruit is a small, affordable, but joyful adventure that you not only can have, but *should* have every morning. And if you pay close attention to it, fruit will help rekindle your sense of wonder and connection to the natural world.

"From a purely hedonistic perspective, walking makes you feel terrific, and you can gain that feeling very quickly."

Chapter Seven

WALK, WALK, WALK
AROUND THE BLOCK

Walking has been called "the ugly duckling of fitness" because it isn't fast or technology-driven—because it doesn't involve sleek clothing—because it isn't the favorite training regimen of major athletes and well-known celebrities. In the meantime, this form of exercise has quietly become America's favorite path to fitness, with more than 17 million frequent participants.

WHY WALKING?

The reasons for walking's popularity are many. Walking is easy, simple, inexpensive and accessible. Most of all, it's extremely effective. This activity is what the forces of evolution designed the human body to do. It is the type of exercise that people are most likely to stay with.

Walking is also a very effective way to reduce stress. It allows a breeze to blow through your mind to loosen the knots of all your problems. If the benefits of exercise could be put into a pill, the resulting product would soon become the most widely-prescribed medication on the market.

A major study found that women who walk briskly for a half hour on most days have lower risks in all the major degenerative disease categories, including stroke, heart disease, cancer, diabetes, osteoporosis and arthritis. These women were better able to control their weight, and they had a reduced incidence of depression.

Perhaps you've heard similar information many times before and you're still not walking. Here's the real reason you might want to develop the habit. From a purely hedonistic perspective, it makes you feel terrific and you can get that feeling very quickly.

In addition, recent studies show that a much greater number of new cells are created in the brains of those who exercise than in the brains of those who don't. This is yet another reminder that even mild exercise can be a very important thing to do.

There's nothing you have to learn to engage in walking. In saying that, I don't make light of the enormous efforts of those who, as a result of accidents, illness or disabilities, have to relearn walking. However, for most of us, the awkward phase on this physical activity is, gratefully, long past. Still you might want to refine your technique.

GETTING STARTED

As with any exercise, you should check in with your doctor before beginning a new walking program. If you're not in the habit of exercising, your physician may have some recommendations on how to gradually build up. If you have joint or back problems, you may want to consult with a physical therapist or a physiatrist (a doctor of physical medicine and rehabilitation) to correct any gait or posture problems. Information on the physiatrists' association is listed in Resources. Or you might call your county medical association to find one. Physical therapists often work in conjunction with orthopedic surgeons.

Otherwise, just stand up straight for your stroll, with a slight forward lean. Walk at a comfortable pace, look ahead, and gradually speed up as you warm up. Then pretend you're in a bit of a hurry, as if you're five minutes late for a meeting. Step onto the heel and roll forward up onto your toes—then push off.

If you want more of a workout, instead of allowing your arms to hang and swing naturally, bend your arms to ninety-degree angles and use them to pump up your walking. This is greatly facilitated by listening to music.

On the slight chance that you haven't tried one while exercising, it's absolutely true that a Walkman playing your favorite upbeat music can take a lot of the drudgery out of walking. MP3 players are tiny and light, and if you're computer savvy, you can find a lot of songs to download from the web. Cassette players are now unbelievably cheap and the personal, portable CD players have come down in price, too.

A MORNING WALKING ROUTINE

If you're not in the habit of walking, or if you don't have a dog, an early morning walk may not seem like an easy routine to establish. But once you try it for a while and experience the pleasure walking imparts to the first part of your day, you'll see it's a very hedonistic thing to do. This activity helps to energize you throughout the day as well.

To make an early morning walk happen easily, take your designated sweats out the night before and place them on a chair or even on top of your socks and sneakers on the floor by the bed. Then you can just pull on your sweats without a lot of effort. Don't tell yourself that you have to have caffeine first, because then you're liable to get into reading the newspaper or finding other distractions. (You can let the coffee brew while you walk.) The truth is that walking—by causing your blood to circulate more quickly—will awaken you in much the same way caffeine does. Caffeine speeds up circulation by causing the blood vessels to constrict. Unfortunately, caffeine also creates a load on your adrenal glands. Walking does not.

There's no need to worry about how you look when you go out for a morning walk. You probably won't see anyone you know, and if you do, they'll be impressed by your being out and about, regardless of how you look. Besides, it's hard not to have a pleasant countenance and rosy cheeks during an early walk, making it more likely that anyone who sees you will think you look great.

Morning walks allow you to participate in the newness of the day. The grass is dewy. Birds are singing. You feel such cool, sweet air on your face. I tell you, it's gourmet air! If this air could be packaged, they'd be selling it the way they sell bottled water.

Even with a few dillydallies to smell flowers, one can have a nice little walk in 15 minutes. This is certainly enough to get the blood circulating and to clear the grogginess of an early morning out of your system in a most gentle manner.

A nice residential area has all sorts of visual appeal on a morning walk, but there are lots of interesting things to note in an urban environment, too. There are early morning deliveries, bakery and coffee aromas, birds, squirrels and the gradual transformation of a community that slumbers into a city that bustles.

Morning seems to me to be a great time to listen to the birds talk. And bird-watching is at its best in these early hours. However, this hobby might be habit-forming, and

THE WEEKLY 100

Recent studies show that only 100 minutes of walking a week imparts significant health benefits. At 17 minutes a day, times 6 days, you're over that 100-minute mark and can still have a day off for good behavior!

One hundred minutes a week is not a huge time commitment. And walking requires no special equipment or clothing. Most people already have athletic shoes and appropriate clothing in their closets. There are no memberships to buy—and there are no young, flat-bellies to make you feel self-conscious.

then you'll begin to competitively count species, reciting their names and other impressive knowledge concerning range and breeding habits. It's a wholesome activity but it gradually requires investments in binoculars, bird books and travel. (The Healthy Hedonist applauds hobbies that involve travel.)

If just appreciating the day isn't enough to keep you from becoming bored, there are lots of other things that can be accomplished during early morning strolls. A low-key study of landscape design can be accomplished, mostly by just observing what your neighbors are doing.

Critical analysis of house paint colors can be conducted. This is an especially useful aesthetic to pursue if your own house will soon need new paint.

Photography is enjoyable in the early morning, too. Black and white photography is well-suited to an early morning urban or rural environment. If any sort of health-oriented pitch fails to motivate you, photography could be just the excuse you need to get up and out early, giving a sort of artistic imperative to the whole endeavor. It will also naturally lead you in new directions on your morning walks, thereby preventing boredom with either the walk or the camera subjects.

WALKS AT OTHER TIMES

There are lots of places to choose for your strolls throughout the course of a day. This is one of the great characteristics of walking—it is infinitely variable by changing the place where you meander. It will never become boring if you just give yourself the opportunity to visit new places. This might be easier to accomplish on the weekend.

But on a weekday, there are convenient ways to fit in some walking. Deliberately parking at the outer edges of shopping center parking lots is one strategy. Refusing to pay for parking lots is another. It means you have to find a spot on the street and walk the rest of the way to your destination. Taking the stairs at work is yet another approach. Stopping occasionally at different parks on your way home can provide inspiration for more random walks.

An evening walk can also be nice, especially after dinner. It's very good for the digestion. And this is a lovely time to chat. In fact, evening walks can be one of the most romantic and relationship-building activities you could pick. Each of you can process the elements of the day. The two of you might discuss pending decisions, or just quietly enjoy the evening and each other's presence.

Photography as an excuse for walking can take you on nice weekend hikes, as you search out interesting parts of town, and beauty in the parks and wild areas near you.

To extend this rationale a bit, with any luck, there's a photo lab within walking distance of your home or work, so you can also get in some strolls while taking film in to be developed, as well as when picking it up. Obviously if you have a digital camera, you won't do this, but in my opinion, using a digital camera isn't nearly as much fun as the anticipation and then thrill of seeing how the film photos have turned out.

INCLEMENT WEATHER EXERCISE STRATEGIES

Whatever you currently think of the idea of a morning walk, I know that the prospects of it are slim once the weather turns either too hot, too cold, too wet or too snowy. So what does a healthy hedonist do then? Believe it or not, we visit the local mall—not to shop, but to walk.

Mall walking is becoming very popular. Small wonder, when malls offer security, pay phones, bathrooms, beverages, companionship and window shopping, as well as perfect "weather" 12 months a year. Many malls have organized walking programs. Call your local mall's administrative office to find out if it has one. If not, you could start a walking group with a friend or two. It might be easier to walk before stores open, but any time is better than none.

If you already started walking before the weather turned bad, you might be ready to *join a gym*, *take dancing classes*, *learn t'ai chi*, or *swim in a heated pool* with adult-only hours. The stairs at the office might become more appealing. A rebounder in the den could also be the answer. (These trampoline-like devices are highly recommended for stimulating the lymph system, which you'll learn more about in the next chapter.)

There is recent research showing that only ten minutes on *a stationary bike*, two or three times a day, can impart major benefits. In terms of time and attention span, this is definitely in the category of minor commitments. Ten minutes on a bike is something you can accomplish while the coffee is brewing.

I find, however, that one of the major problems with stationary bikes for inclement conditions is where to put them. I hate the way they look, and unless you have really huge closets, or space to spare in your bedroom, they're out in the middle of a room. I can't imagine wanting to have one cluttering up the den, but that's just my opinion. The bikes work for two friends of mine. I believe that both friends watch TV and read the paper while biking. You could certainly test the concept on a used stationary bike, because they are easily available in thrift shops and through *Recycler*-type classified ads.

If you decide that a stationary bike would work for you, an investment in a magnetic "trainer"—a device that allows you to use a regular bicycle as a stationary bike—may be warranted. The good thing about the magnetic trainer is that it is small enough to store under a bed or in a closet. (See Resources.)

Jumping rope is one of the most efficient forms of aerobic exercise. You can get your heart rate up really quickly that way. However, if you're truly out of shape, don't work too hard! Actually, that's unlikely, because it takes some practice to get to the point of skillfully coordinating the rope and the footwork. By that time, you're already in much better shape. If jumping rope sounds way too intense, the selling point is that it's cheap, the "equipment" is easy to store, and you can take the rope with you anywhere.

THE UPS & DOWNS OF MY FITNESS JOURNEY

In presenting these ideas about exercise, let me assure you that I'm not a jock. I will not expound at great length on that, but I will merely tell you that my poor eye-hand coordination always made me one of the last chosen for sports teams in high-school physical education (PE) classes. These experiences were excruciating for me and one of the first joys of adulthood was to have reached the point where I no longer had to take a PE class.

But I was never weak. I have a limber, well-constructed frame that was strengthened by ballet lessons (at which I was also rather mediocre), Pilates-based training (which is fabulously effective) when I could afford it, and yoga steadily, if not daily, over the past 22 years. And in the past year, I got back to a more aerobic type of exercise.

My recent return to aerobic exercise happened very gradually. I joined a gym because I wanted access to a sauna, and I thought I might as well work out a bit on the treadmill. Six or seven months later, I paid for some sessions with a trainer, which was a brilliant move on my part. He and I worked out a high-protein vegan diet, and I lost over ten pounds. I started converting middle-age flab back to muscle. Of course, I've gained some of it back while writing this book. It's those minor anxiety attacks that cause me to seek solace with a handful of chocolate chips. Okay, so when I get the book done, I'll quit buying them. The way I see it, it could be worse. But carrot sticks rarely fill the anxiety void the way a little chocolate does.

POETRY IN MOTION

There's lots of information available if and when you're ready to tackle walking more seriously. But as the purpose of this book is to encourage you to tackle activities hedonistically, I'll take another tack. I'd like to suggest a unique way to change the quality of your walks and to fill them with renewable interest and beauty. That is to memorize poetry during your stroll.

Poetry volumes are usually very thin, or a single poem can be photocopied and carried. Those with meter and rhyme can actually help your walking rhythm, the same way music with a beat does. Once the poem is memorized, it's yours to keep for as long as your brain holds out, which will be longer if you exercise.

Poetry is low in calories, but high in nourishment to the soul. I mention this, not only because I love poetry, but also because walking lends itself to all sorts of contemplation, including prayer. In fact, *prayer walking* is becoming a spontaneous, grassroots, leader-less trend. There are a couple of books out on the subject. (See Resources.) If you have trouble staying awake or focused while meditating, prayer walking is a great alternative.

Chapter Eight

BETTER SHOWERING:
MAKING THE MOST OF A GOOD THING

I know that most people already derive tremendous therapeutic benefit from their morning showers. For many, that (and a cup of coffee) is truly what wakes them up.

What would life be like without hot showers? We recently had some plumbing work done at our house, and there was no hot water for two days. It seemed longer. I could have gone to the gym, but I didn't have any meetings scheduled. So for the sake of convenience, I just took sponge baths for the duration. But within minutes after the plumbers left, I was in the shower. I'm sure most of you have had similar experiences while camping or traveling. Well, this experience renewed my "attitude of gratitude" regarding hot water and indoor shower facilities. I do not take them for granted!

A PRE-SHOWER PRACTICE

I invite you to try something new to make your morning shower even more invigorating and useful. I'd like to build your curiosity about it by saying that this is one of the most amazingly simple, yet pleasurable things you can do. It gives you a lovely rush, a tingle, all over your body. And while the practice takes less than a minute to accomplish, it's extremely beneficial. Your investment? A one-time expense of about $7 or $8.

What I'm speaking of is *dry-skin brushing*.

If you go to a health food store, or a large drug store that sells lots of personal care products, you should be able to find a wooden-handled brush with medium-soft bristles of plant origin. If the bristles are too soft, the brushing won't be adequately stimulating. If they're too stiff, brushing will scratch and be irritating. You should find the brushes with the loofah sponges and bath mitts.

You'll find the instructions for this practice in the box labeled "Dry-Skin Brushing, Step by Step."

In addition to being extremely beneficial to your lymph system, which you'll read about soon, this technique also improves the condition of your skin.

THE SKINNY ON SKIN

Here's a little pep talk about skin. Did you know it's the largest organ of your body? Most people don't recognize their skin as such, they just think of organs as being inside the body, something you hope to never see. But your skin actually operates in many ways like your lungs and kidneys. It is entirely permeable. Anything you apply to your skin is absorbed almost immediately into your blood stream. This is how the nicotine patch works. For this reason, it's important to stop buying personal care products that are made with petrochemicals. Chap Stick®? Vaseline®? Baby oil? Look for the vegetable-based equivalents at the health food store and stop rubbing the cosmetic equivalent of motor oil into your skin.

Skin also regulates your body temperature through perspiration. In addition, it has a tremendously important but

DRY-SKIN BRUSHING, STEP BY STEP

When you've undressed, and while you're waiting for the shower to warm up, gently brush your skin toward your heart.

Step 1. Holding the brush in one hand, raise your other arm and begin brushing it from the wrist down to the armpit, going around the arm. This should take about four strokes. Reverse arms and do the same on your other arm.

Step 2. Then start at one ankle and brush up the leg all the way to the groin area. Do this on each leg, addressing all sides, using maybe four strokes to a leg.

Step 3. Now brush up from the waist in front and then very gently around the chest and breasts. Next brush up from the waist in back, as far as you can reach.

Step 4. Brush inward along your collar bone, from the shoulder toward the base of your neck. Do this first on one side, then the other, making four to six strokes on each side.

Step 5. Then brush from the back edge of your shoulder toward the back of your neck, again taking four to six strokes on each side.

Step 6. Next brush down the back of your neck. Now, very, very gently, brush down your cheeks and then back along your jawline toward your neck. Do this on both sides.

little recognized function in detoxification, as do your lungs. Both the skin and the lungs release impurities into the air. But some of those toxins are left on the surface of your skin, along with the salts found in all bodily fluids. That's one of the reasons why after a couple of days without a shower, your skin starts to feel so unpleasant.

Dry-skin brushing benefits your skin in several important ways.

Firstly, you're exfoliating dead skin cells by the mechanics of skin brushing, as well as stimulating both the sweat and oil glands. This not only helps your pores to breathe, it also helps skin to glow. Dead skin cells don't have the luster that living skin cells do.

Secondly, you are, in effect, exercising your skin. The gentle tug of the dry brush across your skin stretches the connective tissues, which stimulates it to renew itself through regeneration of collagen and elastin fibers. In other words, this practice helps your skin stay young-looking. Consistent skin brushing can improve your skin tone and reduce cellulite. It's certainly worth a try, and I'm hoping some of you will report back on your results.

As important as that is for your morale, there's something even more important happening just below the skin. Dry-skin brushing is also one of the easiest, most convenient and most affordable ways to stimulate your lymph system.

Now that I've given you a major hint as to why dry-skin brushing feel so good, let's look a little closer.

A LYMPHATIC SYSTEM PRIMER
The lymphatic system is an essential, but little recognized part of your body's cleansing mechanisms. It partners

and connects with your circulation system, but it has different capabilities and characteristics. Lymphatic fluid is colorless and it surrounds every cell of your body. It is the carrier medium that is used to supply nutrients, which are delivered when elements of the blood pass through the one-cell-thick walls of the capillaries. At this cellular level, nutrients and oxygen are exchanged for carbon dioxide. Then 90 percent of the blood's fluid reenters the bloodstream through the walls of the capillaries and travels back to the heart via the veins. But the 2 to 10 percent that doesn't becomes lymphatic fluid.

As it bathes each individual cell, lymphatic fluid not only delivers nutrients but carries away waste products from the cells, which include excess protein, dead cells, bacteria, viruses, inorganic substances, water and fats. If the skin is properly stimulated, this fluid enters tiny cellular structures called the initial lymphatics, 70 percent of which are located in the skin. The fluid then moves into gradually larger and larger lymphatic vessels until it returns to the bloodstream via the thoracic duct near the heart. On its way, the fluid flows through lymph nodes, where it is cleansed by lymphocytes, the specialized cells that make up one of the most important parts of the body's immune system.

How the lymphatic fluid moves is very interesting. It moves through contractions of the tiny lymph vessels called lymph angions. These have one-way valves that allow the lymphatic fluid to flow only in the general direction of the heart. As each lymph angion swells with lymphatic fluid, its internal sensor tells it to contract, which pushes the fluid forward into the next cell and creates a vacuum effect pulling more fluid up from the lymph angion below.

You are about to understand one of the reasons that

exercise is so incredibly important. What do you suppose causes the lymphatic fluid to move more quickly, which in turn allows toxic by-products to be disposed of more efficiently? As you may have guessed, exercise is one cause. Massage is another. Dry-skin brushing is a third. Inverted yoga postures, such as shoulder stands and head stands, are a fourth. Breathing and the pulsing of arteries also cause this to happen, but not at the more rapid rate.

If your diet is loading your system with excess protein and toxins, and you're not helping the lymphatic fluid to move along with one or more of these methods, the fluid can become like a swamp. The result is sluggishness and fatigue.

This insight into the lymph system tells you why the gentle purposeful strokes of dry-skin brushing help the lymphatic fluid to move up and out, which in turn helps to cleanse your entire body.

Caution: There are a few people who should not do dry-skin brushing. They are those with acute inflammation, malignant tumors, thrombosis or major heart problems. And there are a few people who should check with their licensed health care practitioner before they try it. They are those with kidney problems, bronchial asthma, thyroid problems, persons taking medication or chemotherapy, women who are, or might be, in the first trimester of pregnancy, and those who have had their spleen removed.

For everyone else, this is a very beneficial technique that leaves you tingling all over.

TWO SHOWER STRETCHES

Here's one more way to get a little more energy, a little more renewal, out of that morning shower. These are two

SHAMPOO WITH A NEW TWIST

For a refreshing experience, try adding some essential oils to a fragrance-free shampoo and conditioner that you find at the health food store. Pick something invigorating rather than calming. Besides peppermint oil, other essential oils suggested to give an uplifting effect are sweet basil, orange bergamot, cinnamon, grapefruit, juniper berry, lemon, lime, sweet orange, pine, rosemary, spruce and tangerine. Most of these are listed in the aromatherapy chart included in Chapter 15, "Gifts of the Magi, Gifts for You."

simple yoga stretches you can do right in the shower stall or bathtub. You should use a bathmat or treads in the shower, as slipping there can be dangerous.

An easy way to limber up your back is just to bend over in the shower. Let the hot water hit you right in the lower part of your back. Now hang and breathe.

Breathing releases tension. The way to do this stretch is (rather than struggling to touch your toes) just grab your elbows and breathe. Let the weight of your upper body, the warmth of the shower, and the release of tension that the breathing affords gently stretch out your back a little bit. No exertion is called for. The combination of the three—the weight, the warmth and the breathing will do the work.

If you find water is dripping down into your nose, hold your hands over your face. But concentrate on breathing, not on stretching.

You'll want to balance the exertion to the muscles by doing stretches in one direction first and then the other. So the second stretch is called "a counter stretch." In this move, the counter action is to stretch your arms overhead and then to arch back and breathe.

Naturally, these two stretches can also be done out of the shower. If you have any problems with balance, doing them anywhere other than in the shower is a better idea for you.

FORGET ME NOT

Remembering to do these simple activities is probably the hardest part, especially if you're still not quite awake when you enter the bathroom. You may already be in a hurry to dress and leave for work. Try leaving the dry-skin brush in some obvious spot in the bathroom for a week so that it's hard to miss, or perhaps leave a post-it reminder of the skin brushing and stretching where you'll see it before you turn on the shower. That way, a new habit will begin to form.

"The body needs protein early in the day and carbohydrates at night. This runs counter to how most people eat."

Chapter Nine

REDISCOVERING ENERGY

A couple of years ago, I consulted with a naturopathic physician (N.D.). I could tell that I was falling into a rut. I didn't seem to have the energy I used to have, and I was consuming too much sugar and caffeine to compensate. Throughout the day, my energy was up and down, up and down, depending on how recently I'd had a cup of coffee and something sweet to go with it.

Her answer was "That's easy to fix." The N.D. told me that she'd helped lots of stressed-out high tech employees in Seattle with the same problem. In a nutshell, she advised me to exercise every day and to eat more protein in the early part of the day.

Granted, it took me a while to make that happen consistently (especially the exercise part), but it really worked. Since then, I've learned why.

DR. BAKER'S CIRCADIAN PRESCRIPTION

The latest information on diet shows that your body needs certain substances to be delivered at certain times of the day for maximum efficiency. The body needs protein early in the day and carbohydrates at night. This runs counter to how most people eat. Most folks are eating carbohydrates such as toast, bagels, muffins or cereal for breakfast, and eating protein in the form of meat, poultry or fish at their evening meal. But according to Sidney MacDonald Baker, M.D., that approach delivers raw materials to the body at the wrong times. The result is a late morning and early afternoon sag that sends us running for caffeine, sugar and more carbohydrates.

Dr. Baker's latest book, *The Circadian Prescription*, is based on the research of Dr. Charles Ehret, among others. These researchers found that our bodies respond to the rhythms of Earth—especially the day-to-night and night-to-day 24-hour cycle. The book's title reflects this knowledge. Webster's *New Collegiate Dictionary* defines "*circadian*" as "being... or occurring in approximately 24-hour periods or cycles."

"While we are all different biochemically and deserve custom tailoring of our medical treatment, we are all the same rhythmically," writes Dr. Baker. By this, he means that we are all affected, consciously or unconsciously, by the rhythms of Earth, especially the cycle of dark and light we know as night and day.

Dr. Baker continues by saying scientists have learned that many chemical processes in the body occur in narrow time slots. He describes it with the following analogy: "It's as if a certain department, say in your liver, works on a particular chore from 4:00 p.m. to 5:00 p.m. Then the biochemical workers on that chore are told: 'Shop's closed. Go home. Come back tomorrow at 4:00 p.m. Now the guys on the next shift are coming in to do their job.'"

This is one small example of the biological processes that are happening each day at fairly specific times within the body. Dr. Baker calls the need to sleep at night the most obvious one. Humans do better when they're awake during the day and asleep at night.

This physician-author predicts that, in the future, our health and that of our children and grandchildren will be improved by advances in scientific understanding of how the many circadian rhythms of the body can be made more harmonious. He believes the fields of what are being called "*chronobiology*" and "*chronopharmacology*" will teach us to synchronize the intake of various medications, nutrients and other stimuli with the timing of chemical and electrical events in the body.

And what is that timing? According to Dr. Baker, and the research on which his book is based, we should eat the majority of our daily protein intake for breakfast and lunch and eat only carbohydrates for dinner. In his medical practice, he has found this resolves a huge problem that many people have of eating too many carbohydrates too early in the day, which then causes high serum insulin levels, among a long list of other damaging effects.

I've tried it. In the boxed section called "This Healthy Hedonist's Food Plan," you'll find the food sequence that has worked so well for me.

This eating plan separates when you eat proteins and carbohydrates. You don't have to be obsessive about it, but this is a concept described as "food-combining" that takes our biology into account more than most menus do. Actually, it's food un-combining. It's based on the biological fact that our ancestors didn't have the variety of foods that we have available at every meal. Our ancestors pretty much ate one thing at a time. So our digestive processes evolved to digest one type of food at a time. Based on this evolution, protein and carbohydrates require different digestive juices,

THIS HEALTHY HEDONIST'S FOOD PLAN

1. Fruit first. I eat a piece before I go for a walk and have another piece when I come back.

2. Then, a half hour later, I drink a smoothie. A more exact recipe is in the recipe section, but my smoothies are made with a piece or two of fruit, a bit of apple juice and soy protein powder.

3. Mid-morning, I eat either a commercial soy protein bar or one of my homemade ones (which are more nutritious and less costly than the ones you buy). The recipe is in the back of this book.

4. There's more protein at lunch. I usually have homemade bean soups. But then, I'm usually eating lunch at home. If that doesn't work for you, low-fat yogurt is an easy and affordable way to have protein at noon when you're at work. If you go out to lunch, grilled meat, fish or poultry and a salad would be excellent, or if you're a vegetarian like me, a tofu stir fry would work. (I'm not insistent about the protein for lunch at restaurants. I often have a salad or pasta. As you'll see in Chapter 22, "Eating Out & Traveling," I've found ways to blend my dietary preferences into almost all kinds of restaurants.)

5. Mid-afternoon, or on the way home from work, I enjoy an apple, fresh fruit juice or soy nuts. (See Chapter 12, "Home, James!")

6. I eat pasta, potatoes or other carbohydrates at night, along with salad or fresh juice.

On weekends, having eggs or a tofu scramble for breakfast fits well in this plan and provides lots of mental and physical energy.

and those juices, when combined in the stomach, have the effect of canceling each other out. Poor digestion is the result. When you eat protein and carbohydrates separately, your food digests more completely, you derive more nutrition from it, and you experience less bloat.

The glorious thing about this approach is that you don't have to count calories or fat grams and no one's telling you exactly what to eat. You can have a lot of flexibility about the foods you choose. The important thing is when to eat protein and when to eat carbohydrates and that you try not to combine them.

If you want to understand the whole idea more fully, I recommend reading *The Circadian Prescription*. But in the meantime, my suggestion is that you follow The Healthy Hedonist's food plan for a couple of weeks. See how you feel. I believe you'll have more stable energy, less hunger and fewer cravings and you might even lose a couple of pounds.

Now, dear reader, I know there are a lot of skeptics among you. I have tried this way of eating and found it made a huge difference in my energy. This, in turn, made it possible for me to avoid eating so much sugary and starchy food, which was causing me to begin to look like a middle-aged woman.

Now chronologically, I am a middle-aged woman. But I don't think like one, I don't act like one, and it's for damn sure I don't want to look like one—at least not so long as there's something I can to do to prevent it.

My food plan offers enough low-fat protein that, when combined with weight training, you can move toward major improvements to your shape.

A QUICK LOOK AT VEGETARIANISM

I mentioned earlier I'm a vegetarian, but I don't preach about it. Becoming a vegetarian is not about having a religious experience. It's about being healthy, but not at the expense of happiness. If you're not ready for it, vegetarianism won't work for you. It doesn't work for everyone. I've known people who have tried it for years, but found that they weren't able to absorb enough nutrients eating strictly vegetarian. All I can say is that it works for me. My diet evolved and is still evolving. One year, I gave up beef. The next year, I gave up chicken and fish. A few years after that, I gave up dairy. I'm down to a bit of "social" and "traveling" cheese. That's just how I did it. I'm not trying to convince you.

THE SOY SENSATION

I will, however, sing the praises of soy. A soybean is made up of the following nutritional components:

42% protein
33% carbohydrate
20% oil
5% hull

The protein content of products made from soybeans varies, so you'll have to read the label to know the exact percentage. However, it's safe to say that soy offers equivalent protein levels to meat, dairy and eggs, with very little fat and none of the food safety risks associated with animal products (such as trichinosis, mad cow disease, salmonella, e-coli).

Soy is mentioned more and more as one of the most important ways for men and women to help reduce the risk of prostate and breast cancers, respectively. The isoflavones found in soy help the body adjust harmful hormone levels, whether they're high or low.

A study at Loma Linda University found that Seventh Day Adventist men in California who consumed soymilk at least once per day had a 70 percent reduced risk of developing prostate cancer. Another study found similar results for Japanese American men who ate tofu.

Epidemiological studies have shown that women in Asia have lower rates of breast cancer than American women and it is thought to be partly the result of consuming soy.

Soy also helps relieve the effects of menopause. It's been shown to reduce the frequency of hot flashes by as much as 60 percent. Soy offers these benefits at low cost and without the possible negative side effects of estrogen replacement therapies.

Another important benefit of soy is that it seems to prevent osteoporosis. Studies show that one of the nutrients of soy works to help stave off bone deterioration.

Soy also has antioxidant properties that reduce the effect of free radicals, the rogue molecules that damage healthy tissue by stealing electrons. Recent research has shown how important antioxidants are in reducing the effects of aging.*

Some people are allergic to soy, and if it causes your digestive system distress, you might also be allergic to it. You could have an allergy test if you want to be sure, but just watching how your body reacts to it is simpler.

Provided you're not allergic to soy, the benefits of a moderate amount of soy may be too important to overlook. If taste and not knowing how to use soy have been stopping you from incorporating more soy into your diet, you can move ahead now using some of my ideas.

I use soy protein in my smoothie every morning. One serving of soy protein powder gives me 11 grams of protein and 22 mg. of isoflavones for only 55 calories .

I also buy protein bars made with soy protein, as opposed to milk or whey protein. In addition you'll find a recipe for homemade soy protein energy bars among the recipes I've provided. The homemade bars are about half as expensive as buying the most inexpensive bars at stores, and they're more nutritious because of the natural ingredients I've selected. Making the energy bars yourself is a more environmentally sound practice, too—there's no packaging. It takes me about a half hour to make them. The recipe keeps me and my husband supplied with highly nutritious mid-morning snacks for about a week.

In cooking, soy takes on the flavor of whatever it is seasoned with. There are now thousands of products that are made with soy, especially in health food stores, but also a surprising number in regular stores.

There are all sorts of soy burgers, soy hot dogs, soy breakfast sausages, soy pepperoni, soy sandwich slices including bologna as well as "ham" flavor and "turkey" flavors. There are even soy Italian sausages. You can get slivered soy that imitates chicken and beef for use in stir fries. There are also soy-based products to substitute for mayonnaise, sour cream and several of the more commonly used cheeses. In fact, over 2,000 soy products have been created in the past decade.

Lately, quite a number of soy snack products have appeared. This is the fastest growing section of the soy marketplace.

There are lots of ways to go about a soy discovery mission. You could go to your health food store and buy a number of soy snack products all at once, and compare them, side by side. Or you could just try one at a time, maybe one a week. See how the different products go over with the rest of your household.

If your other household members aren't willing to eat soy knowingly, you can start to experiment with disguising them. You can substitute texturized vegetable protein (available at your health food store) in recipes that call for ground beef—in pasta sauce, for example. When you've added spices and given the sauce time to simmer, it's unlikely your household members will be able to tell the difference. Another idea is to use veggie sausages in sauces and casseroles where they can be incorporated very inconspicuously.

With the recent approval by the FDA of cholesterol-lowering claims on the labels of soy products, the creation of new soy choices promises to continue at an even faster pace. This is a good time to begin experimenting. Ask the manager of your health food store for a personal recommendation.

Besides energy bars, other types of soy snack products are compared on the next page.

*See thehealthyhedonist.com for news on recent soy research.

SOY SNACK COMPARISON

Product	Serving Size	Calories Per Serving	Protein Grams Per Serving	Fat Grams Per Serving	Comments
Soy crackers	20 crackers	120	7	2	Wide variety in taste of different brands.
Soy crisps	25 crisps	100	7	2	I like these a lot. Flavors include ranch, barbeque and others.
"Dr. Soy" cookies	4 cookies	170	9	3	Similar to conventional cookies, but more protein. A good mid-morning snack.
Soy trail mix	1 oz.	110	7	4	Comes in various flavors. Tropical blend is sweet enough to satisfy my sweet tooth.
Soy nuts, honey roasted	1/4 cup	130	10	5	Some of my favorite soy munchies.
Soy nuts, barbeque flavor	1/3 cup	130	9	7	Tasty with about half the fat of peanuts.
Organic chocolate soy nuts	1/4 cup	190	7	11	Rather high in fat, but truly a healthy hedonist snack.

"When I have a scheduled meeting, I pile the meeting materials by the door. I have to, because at the last minute, I can barely remember my name."

Chapter Ten

EASY EXITS

MY MORNINGS

Getting out the door on time in the morning has always been problematical for me. I'm talking about the time it takes to pick up my purse, grab a bottle of water, an apple or two and a protein bar to take with me, put on my watch and earrings and paint my nails. (I paint them right before I get into the car, with everything else already in the car and the keys in the ignition. That's the only way I manage to get nail polish to dry without smudging.)

If I'm not careful, I tend to run 10 minutes late for my first appointment of the day, and that's been going on since I was in high school. I remember on numerous occasions in college grinning sheepishly at the professor of my 7:30 a.m. biology class as I tried to slide into my seat after he had already begun the lecture. I can still feel my embarrassment and discomfort at the pained expression he always gave me in return.

I don't have kids to get ready for school. I just have to coordinate schedules with my husband Patrick, contend with the "oh-I-know-you're-about-to-abandon-me-forever" look from my dogs and make sure all the windows and doors are locked.

But I have developed a few helpful habits. I always leave my keys in the same place by the door. My purse is generally over-equipped and ready to go. When I have a scheduled meeting, I pile the meeting materials by the door. I have to, because at the last minute, I can barely remember my name.

By the time you've read this far, you can tell I think a bit of organization allows my mind to wander with fewer negative consequences. My sister always says, "A person with her head in the clouds should keep her shoelaces tied."

EASING YOUR MORNINGS & MORE

If the above ideas or similar strategies would make it easier for you to get out the door in the morning and consequently reduce a.m. stress, it could be well worth the effort to start using them. Let's think about how that could work for you.

Ask yourself the following questions:

1. What always delays you in the morning?
2. What could be done the night before or on the weekend to avoid that?
3. Would it be worthwhile to intrude into your down time to take stress prevention measures?

You are the only person who can answer that last question for yourself. However, my morning sanity is definitely worth taking steps like putting my keys in the same place by the door when I come in. That way, I never have to panic trying to find them. Now I don't even think about this. It's simply something I do automatically.

Creating an outgoing mail basket or box is another good idea. Then the first person out in the morning makes a habit of taking the mail.

Could the preparation of your and/or your family's brown bag lunches be turned into an assembly line? Can assembly of nonperishable items be done on the weekend, with much of the rest of it done the night before?

What about getting dressed? Would it make sense to lay out five outfits on Sunday evening and match them up with all the underwear and accessories they require? You could then put the accessories and underwear in a bag and hang it on the hanger with the clothes. Or try this with just one day's clothes. Would it be worth it to try to get the kids to do this for themselves?

There are ways to make dressing decisions easier. I have concluded that more than to convey a sense of sophistication, the real reason some people often wear black is that all black clothing matches rather well and none of it shows dirt. I had always thought that black was too severe a color for me. However, when I gave in to making it the foundation color of my wardrobe, dressing became ten times easier. My uniform is black pants or skirt, white shirt and whatever jacket seems appropriate. With slight variations, this is how I dress 80 percent of the time I go out.

Besides black and white, navy with either tan or khaki is another classic color combination. In the summer, beige and white looks very sharp. Using a couple of these basic color schemes can also facilitate business travel. It makes shopping much easier as well, since there's less to worry about in coordinating colors. If the colors seem boring to you, use accessories to liven them up.

If you discovered this ages ago and have more great tips you've discovered since, please email them to me at janet@thehealthyhedonist.com.

What about non-regular details that need to be taken care of before you leave the house the next morning? Do permission slips need to be signed? Do bills and other stuff need to be mailed the next day? Can you eliminate those details the night before so that everything you have to think about before you leave the next morning has already been done? Incidentally, if you have problems sleeping, this can be another way to help relieve the anxiety that is keeping you awake.

I know from my own life that it's not possible to devote every night to stress reduction. There are classes to attend, bill payments that need to go out, magazines and newspapers to read, email to answer, dishes and laundry to be done, phone calls to return, and activities that need to be set up. It never ends. Leaving it all to be done over the weekend might mean there won't be time for much fun on the weekend and that's not a good idea either.

But in terms of a strategy for sanity, can mid-week chores be grouped into certain nights—leaving other nights relatively free? Can you arrange your weekly schedule so that not every evening is spent dealing with the overflow of details that merely get you from one day to the next with no actual break in the stress you experience at work? Can you carve out one or two nights during the week when you concentrate on relaxing and pampering yourself with light eating, walking, bathing (and the other forms of active relaxation you'll read about in subsequent chapters)? Can you postpone bills, email, voice mail, newspapers, magazines and other potentially disturbing sources a couple of nights a week? Or at least after a certain time of night, say 9 p.m.?

WHAT'S AT STAKE

The big underlying issue here is boundaries. Whose life is it, anyway? Don't you have the right to enjoy some of the time during the week in activities that are intrinsically pleasurable, not just getting you home and ready to come back to work again the next day?

I think the answer is an emphatic *yes!*, but how we answer that question in our own lives is different for each of us.

"Work is an essentioal part of being alive. Your work is your identity. It tells you who you are. It's gotten so abstract. People don't work for the sake of working. They're working for a car, a new house, or a vacation. It's not the work itself that's important to them. There's such a joy in doing work well."

Kay Stepkin

"The ability to keep your perspective in a high-pressure environment and to enjoy most work days without becoming overwhelmed is a learned skill. "

Chapter Eleven

WORK IN BALANCE

Surfing is a good analogy for the successful handling of career pressures. One wants to ride the wave at work, as opposed to swallowing sea water, getting hit in the head by the surfboard or, worst case, drowning. Surfing is a learned skill. It requires strength, balance and perseverance. Few people are able to ride a surfboard the first time they try. Similarly the ability to keep your perspective in a high-pressure environment, to enjoy most workdays without becoming overwhelmed, is also a learned skill. And because work stress affects your capacity to enjoy life when you're not at work, "work surfing" is definitely a skill you'll want to master as a healthy hedonist.

There are seven areas to be considered. For your ease of use, I've divided these areas into two groups —small steps and large steps.

The small steps are much easier. Like many of the other suggestions in this book, they can give you more energy to tackle the larger steps. The small steps include:

- Enhancing your workspace
- Establishing better health habits at work
- Utilizing emergency stress measures

The big steps are very personal in nature and have to be

worked through over a period of time. However, when you're really ready, you may be able to move through these large steps very quickly.

- Defining your goals and values
- Visualizing successful outcomes
- Learning conflict resolution and how to deal with difficult personalities
- Mastering organizational techniques

ENHANCING YOUR WORKSPACE

The comments in this section are addressed to those of you who work in offices. If you don't work in an office, skip ahead to the healthy habits section, which applies to everyone.

PERSONAL TOUCHES

Most people have permission to personalize their office spaces, and it's an important option. If you have a supportive work environment, where the efforts of team members are regularly and enthusiastically recognized, you may not have as great a need for an identity "bubble" at your desk. But if your work environment is not particularly supportive, having reminders of the people who love you and items that reflect who you really are can be extremely important. In moments of stress, you can draw strength from these sources.

Most people have photos of their children or spouse in their workspace. But this idea can be expanded. What are your goals? To buy your dream house? To move to a quiet place in the country? To send your child to a great school? Perhaps you can find a picture to remind you of a larger lifetime goal. It could also be a photo of a person you admire and want to emulate.

Another important item for your workspace is a photo of you having fun, possibly on your most recent vacation, or at a party, or just at home doing what you most love to do. Your calm, relaxed self is your true self. Don't allow job stress to distort who you are.

PLANTS

Besides photographs and mementos, I strongly suggest a plant or two. Plants in general provide a bit of nature, as well as cleaning the air through their respiration processes. Some have the ability to absorb toxins! Two of the plants recommended most often for that purpose are spider plants, technically known as *Chlorophytum bichetii* and *Chlorophytum comosum*. They're attractive and easy to maintain.

A weekly investment in a rose or a small bouquet of flowers can brighten your office and create enjoyment for you and your coworkers. The color and beauty that flowers provide is one of those little hedonistic things that feeds your soul. Unlike choices in music or aromatherapy, which might not coincide with everyone else's tastes, it's unusual to find a flower that other people don't like. Buying flowers every week is a way of telling yourself, "I'm worth it. I deserve pleasure."

SOOTHING MUSIC

The ability to calm oneself is an important skill in today's work environment. Otherwise it's difficult to be consistently creative. I find that certain low-tone classical music, such as a solo cello piece, is helpful to me when I'm trying to calm down and process a pile of work. If your office environment allows you to play quiet music, it can be very soothing. There are many kinds of healing music now available that would also be appropriate. (See Resources.)

FOUNTAINS

A little fountain is a nice way to enhance your office, and these accessories are now very affordable. Running water also creates negative ions, which are said to stimulate creativity. Fountains are also a nice reminder of nature. The sound of a "babbling brook" reaches us at an unconscious level. It's a calming, peaceful addition to your work environment.

BETTER HEALTH HABITS AT WORK

One of the benefits of implementing healthy hedonism in your life away from the office is that some of those habits will automatically spill over to your hours at work. Nevertheless, your health habits at the office do deserve some specific attention.

EATING DURING THE WORKDAY

The question of what to eat throughout the workday is a challenge. In this effort, the following thoughts could be helpful.

Being both thrifty and health conscious, I've always found that bringing "lunch and munch" provisions with me is a good way to save money and eat smarter. It always surprises me what people will spend on food of poor nutritional quality. I know that bringing a lunch to work is not a hip thing to do. Perhaps people feel it doesn't fit their image, or they're just too busy in the morning to bother with packing a lunch. To make packing a "brown bag" easier, I suggest that you incorporate an office lunch category into the weekly shopping. Buy things that don't require refrigeration. It gives you something to fall back on when you're too busy to go out for lunch. If you have a credenza or a spare drawer, perhaps you can just keep a few items on hand. It sure beats having fast food ordered in. I've made a few suggestions below as to what your list might include, but there are dozens of possibilities.

Fruit for mid-morning and mid-afternoon snacks is a primary suggestion. If you have a spot in your office where you can place a fruit bowl, you could bring a week's worth on Monday and enjoy it all week long as a decorative element, as well as a snack bar. It's even possible that an office fruit bowl could work as a cooperative venture for the greater health and aesthetic pleasure of all!

Commercial *energy bars* can be extremely helpful. If you buy them by the box, you can bring the cost down by 10 to 20 percent. Even at a couple dollars a day, these are certainly a better health investment than expensive coffee drinks. Some of the energy bars are more nutritious than others. They're definitely worth experimenting with. Snacks are important to keep your blood sugar up, but resorting to nutritionally deficient candy bars, cookies and other pastries should be the exception rather than the rule.

I've included a recipe for homemade bars in the recipe section. (See "JB's Energy Bars.") Bringing these in on a weekly basis and storing them in a plastic container in the office refrigerator is something to consider. (If your office mates find out how delicious they are, you might have to make sure no one can tell what's in the container, otherwise they may mysteriously disappear.) More energy bar recipes are available on our website, *www.thehealthyhedonist.com.*

While I'm not a big fan of sandwiches, I'm also not a nut about avoiding them. I just happen to think of sandwiches as flawed in terms of optimal eating. You read about food combining in Chapter 9, "Rediscovering Energy." Although sandwiches are a very portable and convenient food, they're examples of poor food combining, as they almost inevitably combine protein (meat) and carbohydrates (bread) at the same meal. Hamburgers and other fast food sandwiches have the same inherent problem, and they are usually high in saturated fat. So as a lunch option, sandwiches should be an exception rather than the rule.

What would I recommend eating for lunch? If you're not opposed to bringing in "*planned-overs*" from home and heating them in the office microwave there are a lot of possibilities. Invest in ceramic food storage containers if you're heating your food in plastic containers. The heat of the microwave causes molecules from the plastic to migrate into your food, creating cancer-causing dioxins. The health ramifications could be nasty.

When you don't have suitable planned-overs, *a yogurt-based lunch* is a good option, with smoothies being just one possibility. These lunches are affordable, offer protein that will stay with you and also provide "*probiotics.*" These are the friendly intestinal bacteria such as *Lactobacillus acidophilus* that have the ability to significantly enhance one's digestion.

There are a lot of possibilities on how to prepare the yogurt. You could mix it with fresh fruit and fruit juice to make a nutritious smoothie. Granola or other forms of cereal can be added, as well as crunchy and nutritious ingredients such as raw sunflower or pumpkin seeds. Experiment until you find a combination you enjoy.

To derive the most benefit from a yogurt lunch, don't purchase the sugary yogurt products you find in the supermarket. Buy high-quality plain yogurt from a health food store and look on the label to see that it has "live cultures." This means the bacteria has not been killed through a pasteurization process.

You might not want to eat yogurt every day for lunch, but a couple of times a week it can be an affordable, convenient and highly nutritious lunch or mid-morning snack.

In terms of restaurant lunch options, look for places near your work that make *homemade soups* or *Asian foods*. These are options that are affordable on a daily basis, as well as nutritionally sound. At Asian restaurants, avoid deep fried items and eat plenty of vegetables and some steamed rice. (Ask if they have brown rice.) Also, request that no MSG be used in cooking your order.

If you can find a place that serves *fresh salads*, you could improve the taste and nutritional benefit by compiling a healthy salad condiment kit, as described more fully in Chapter 22, "Eating Out & Travel." The condiment kit is something you would carry in to a fast food restaurant to dress up the salads available there. It's also something you can leave in your desk; then you could bring the salads back and dress them up with your personal stash of salad goodies.

BEVERAGES

A decent cup of coffee at work is important. But most of us have better places to spend our money than paying somewhere between $4 and $8 a day for coffees from a commercial establishment selling fancy versions of java. (The math is easy. At $4 a day, it's an expenditure of $20 a week, or $80 a month, which would easily pay for a very pleasant evening out.) The way around this is to create a small and inexpensive coffee setup at work. This can easily be done by bringing pre-ground coffee in an air-tight container to the office or even buying a grinder and grinding the coffee at work. The approach is still cheap compared to buying expensive coffees day after day. Then use either a French press or a tiny Melita filter and cone to make an individual cup of high-quality coffee (however strong you like it). You could use boiling hot water from an electric kettle that can serve both the drip coffee and tea needs of the entire office. (Electric kettles only cost about $30, and you could probably raise the money through office donations, or talk the boss into spending this amount. Tell the boss that this one-time expenditure will not only boost morale, but will save the 15 minutes or more that people take to go out to buy coffee.)

In addition to monetary benefits and productivity improvements by staying closer to your desk, there are a few health benefits that can be derived by making your own caffeinated beverages at the office. One is that you can then purchase organic coffees and teas. Also, you can use better water than what comes out of the tap. According to my investigations, the expensive commercial coffee establishments are using tap water, not filtered.

Your most healthful beverage choices are plain, filtered water or herb teas. You might try to develop a habit of drinking a detox tea once a day at work. (See Chapter 23, "Maximum Fun, Minimum Damage.") One way I've found to make water more interesting is to top it off with a commercial blend of cranberry and raspberry juice. Adding fresh lemon juice is very beneficial if you like the flavor.

STRETCHING AT WORK

There are a couple of yoga and other stretches that can easily be done at the office. Our bodies were designed to move, not stay in the same position hour after hour. A stretch break every couple of hours is time well spent.

Spinal Twist in a Chair

This is a wonderful way to loosen the lower back where we accumulate so much stress. Do it in any chair that has a back of sufficient height to allow you to drape your arm over it.

1. With your feet on the floor in front of you, straighten your left arm and place it on the outside of your right knee.
2. Inhale, and then as you exhale, gradually and gently twist to the right, allowing your right elbow to drape over the top of the chair back.
3. Then with your eyes closed, breathe in. Without straining, use your exhalation to twist just a tiny bit further. Breathe in and out several times, and each time you exhale, twist a little tiny bit further, but do this very gently. Don't strain. Don't pull.
4. Gradually attempt to look over your shoulder. Lead with your eyes, looking behind you.
5. Then gently unwind and reverse the pose, turning in the other direction and following the same steps.

Other Stretches

Hunch up your shoulders and roll them a couple of times each way (to the front and then to the back). Next, wiggle your shoulders and your torso, moving all the way down to your hips. Then, shake out your hands. Finally, stretch your neck forward and back, left and right, and then all around in a big circle, first in one direction, then the other direction.

The upcoming forward bend is discussed again in Chapter 17, "A Time of Peace," where you'll find illustrations of each position. However it's a good one to do a couple of times a day at the office.

1. Stand up, with your feet slightly spread. Inhale and then stretch your hands out overhead.

2. Exhale and bend forward from the hips.

3. When you've bent over as far as you naturally can, grab your elbows, let your neck and shoulders relax, and just breathe. Let the weight of your upper body stretch out your back. Keep your knees straight, but not locked. Don't bounce. Don't pull. Just breathe for at least 10 to 15 seconds.

4. Stretch out your arms, clasp your hands, and inhale as you rotate back to an upright position from the hips. Let your eyes follow your hands upward, until your hands are straight up in the air and you're looking up at them.

5. Keep your arms outstretched overhead. While continuing to watch your hands, exhale as you arch your back by gently thrusting your hips forward. Try to keep your arms up and alongside your ears as you bend back. Breathe a couple of times in this position. Then return to an upright position, eyes forward. Allow your arms to relax back at your sides.

EYE RELAXATION

Now give your eyes a moment of rest. First rapidly rub the heels of your palms together until you generate heat. Then place the heels of your hands over your eyes and take a moment to breathe. Don't press on your eyes.

ERGONOMICS

If you're spending most of your day at a computer terminal, having an ergonomically correct chair, mouse and mouse pad can all be tremendously important to reducing stress and protecting your health. If you wear prescription glasses, the purchase of a set of glasses for use specifically at the computer can reduce eyestrain. A glare guard on the monitor can also help.

Hopefully your boss is enlightened, the company is doing well, and you're regarded as indispensable. Then you may be able to persuade the company to purchase a good chair, along with an ergonomically shapped mouse and mouse pad for your use. Relative to workers' compensation costs, the mouse and pad are very inexpensive. A chair can be depreciated. Talk to the bookkeeper.

If the boss won't buy you the chair that's best for your back, think about how much time you spend in that chair and how important good support is to your health. It's like a good bed. No matter how much money you spend on it, when you amortize the price over the number of days you'll use the bed, this is a small cost relative to the benefit it provides. Back problems can definitely interfere with your enjoyment of life. Take care of your back!

If you spend a lot of time on the phone, you should get a headset rather than cradling the phone between your ear and your shoulder.

EMERGENCY STRESS MEASURES

Stress relief is a pillar of healthy hedonism, and this book is packed with various ways to reduce stress throughout the day. Many of them deal with your body's biochemical ability to process stress hormones. Those are the ongoing techniques you need to incorporate. But on an emergency basis, what can you do to relieve stress quickly?

One way is to breathe. Yoga breathing is the fastest, most discreet way to blow off excessive stress. What I'm about to present is a very powerful yoga breathing technique that can rapidly increase the amount of oxygen in your entire bloodstream. It has an immediate calming effect.

But it's also important to remind you how oxygen relates to physical vitality. On a cellular level, energy is released when the mitochondria convert oxygen and glycogen to create adenosine triphosphate (ATP). Without either oxygen or glycogen, you have no energy. It's the same in your body as in your car. Oxygen must be present for fuel to burn and energy to be released. This is just one of the reasons that good posture at your desk is important. If you're slumped over, your lungs cannot expand as much.

BELLOWS BREATH
1. Take a medium-sized breath.
2. With your mouth closed, forcibly expel the air through your nose with a quick snort. Notice how your abdomen makes a rapid contraction, and then expands again with the involuntary breath you take following the snort. That quick exhalation and the involuntary breath that follows are the essence of this breathing technique.

3. Next try a rapid series of five of these breaths.
4. Then expel all the air in your lungs and take a long deep breath.
5. Hold this breath for seven to ten seconds. Then gently release that breath.
6. Repeat this series three times. Gradually increase the number of rapid breaths, and then the length of time that you hold the long breath.

The Bellows Breath is a good way to relieve stress when you're going into an important meeting, when you have to prepare for a difficult conversation, before you speak in front of a group or in any situation that makes you stressed or nervous. It's something you can do in the car while driving, especially when you're stressing out in traffic. It's so simple that you may not yet believe how powerful it can be. If you can't get the hang of it, look in the Yellow Pages for a yoga school. They'll be able to teach this to you, along with a lot of other great stress reduction techniques.

If you worry that someone passing your cubicle door will hear you doing Bellows Breath, I recommend that you go outside for a brief period to do it. In fact, I strongly believe in going outside at least a couple of times a day, even if it's only for five minutes. The air, hopefully a bit of a breeze, can adjust your perspective quite effectively. It's sort of like a smoking break, but instead it's a breathing break.

This is especially important if you work in a sealed office building. The indoor air quality in office buildings is notoriously bad because, in most cases, it's all recirculated. There are a lot of pollutants inside office buildings—fumes from new carpets, new furniture and toner fluids are at the top of the list, and those toxins just keep recirculating. Plus, molds, allergens, bacteria and viruses circulate within a building's ventilation system. Yes, these can seriously affect your health, but I don't mean to be an alarmist about it. That's why you want toxin-absorbing spider plants in your office. But here I just want to emphasize a couple of the reasons why it's important to get outside to breathe. If you can find a spot near work where there are trees and birds, you can also reconnect with nature.

In 1943, Abraham Maslow, the famous psychiatrist of the mid-20th century, first published his concept of a "hierarchy of needs." On the bottom were physiological needs, such as food. Next came safety needs that would be provided by secure shelter. After that came the belongingness and love needs, and so on, up the pyramid to self-actualization and transcendence. When we compare our day-to-day problems at work with Maslow's hierarchy of needs, our problems generally are "higher level" complaints. Except for a small percentage of individuals in the developed world, our most basic needs will usually be covered. We're working toward self-actualization and the other intangible needs ranked higher on the pyramid.

So a breathing break can be used to remind oneself, "Well, this (whatever the problem-of-the-day is) is a nice problem to have." And what would a solution look like? With a fresh supply of oxygen and a quick adjustment to your sense of where an immediate problem fits into the Big Picture, it is possible to return to the office with an attitude that says, "I am renewed."

I do not mean to imply that problems at work are trivial. I know they can even intrude on your nights and weekends, if you let them. But I also know that it's impossible to find real solutions when one is seething with anger and resentment, or on the verge of panic caused by an overload of work that's been dumped on your desk. So any way one can find to quickly get out from under such emotions is a very positive step toward overcoming the associated problem.

And on days when you can't take even ten minutes to go outside for a breathing break, take a one-minute rest. Take a deep breath and hold it for as long as possible. When you release it, visualize your stress and anxiety blowing out with the exhaled air.

GOALS & VALUES

Yogi Berra, the famous catcher and later coach for the New York Yankees said it best. "You've got to be careful if you don't know where you're going, because you might not get there."

A large part of feeling good at work is having a sense of how your job fits into your life goals and your larger sense of purpose. If your job is just a way to pay the bills, that's okay—so long as the job leaves you with enough time and energy at the end of the day or the week to do the things you really want to do.

Your personal values and ethics are also important. It's very stressful to work in an environment where you feel that your values are being compromised. This is especially true if the work you are asked to do does not coincide with what you believe is right. This is not to say I think anyone should quit on the spot. But finding a place to work where the values coincide with your own will give you energy you didn't know you had.

The process of determining goals and values is as varied as there are people. You may know in a flash what they are. Or you may need years of personal introspection to sort them out. But sort them out you must if you wish to be a fulfilled and happy person. I encourage you to openly express your values at your place of work. If enough smart, energetic and intelligent people do so (which is to say, the people on whom the success of any company depends), then there is hope for a better world.

VISUALIZATION & AFFIRMATIONS

Our subconscious mind does not know the difference between "reality" and a well-imagined visualization. Self-improvement experts, spiritual masters, and athletic trainers all encourage visualization to see, hear and feel the desired outcome, which then becomes something the subconscious works to bring into reality. Affirmations can also help you to manifest your goals into reality. With repetition, they imprint a declaration of progress on the subconscious that provides a counterweight to the frustrations of daily life. The affirmations will instill the determination to keep making the concrete incremental steps that move you forward toward your goals.

Learning to be positive is part of the journey many of us must make as adults. The media often glamorize young entertainers who are cool, hip and cynical. Young people emulate such entertainers and think they are to be admired. The opposite is true, but it can take some years of living to figure that out. As an adult, I've grown into the realization that it takes courage to be positive, to plan and project and to move ahead to bring positive goals into reality. Visualization is part of that process. Let it work for you.

CONFLICT RESOLUTION

We spend more time with people at work than we spend during waking hours with our families. Inevitably, points of contention arise. With so much time spent together, and with so much external pressure to succeed, learning how to respond to comments from people with problem personalities at work is an extremely important skill to develop. It has taken me too many years to realize that we don't have to just "take it" from coworkers and/or bosses, suppress the emotions their comments provoke, and then try to emotionally adjust to an insult in the hours outside of work.

This is not to say that you can reactively explode either. What you need to be able to do is respond in a calm, deliberate manner that demonstrates you're a person who won't be taken advantage of.

Learning how to appropriately respond to issues that arise truly can make a stronger, more productive team. It can also help tremendously in one's personal life.

A number of books, tapes, videos and seminar products teach these skills, and I've listed some of them in the Resources Section. Maybe you can persuade your boss to pay for seminars on these subjects, because it benefits more than just your own working environment. It's also a good way to meet other businesspeople in your community who are tackling similar personal and professional issues. If you're not able to attend seminars, your local library probably has materials on these subjects. Books and tapes can be extremely valuable in enhancing your self-esteem. Then it becomes a matter of practice. It's back to the surfing metaphor. Just keep working on it. As you become stronger and improve your balance, you'll do a better job of staying on the surfboard. And if you fall off, it's no big deal. Just climb right back on and get ready to catch the next wave!

ORGANIZING SYSTEMS

Organizational systems can also be a tremendous tool for relieving office stress. A number of different approaches and systems are available.

My favorite is a system described in detail by David Allen in his book *Getting Things Done, The Art of Stress-Free Productivity*. (An audio version is also available.) Allen's approach provides a concrete way to deal with not just the work-related details that are taking up space in your brain, but also your personal projects. He shows you how to bring both the big projects and all the little details into a reliable system. Allen has perfected his technique over 20 years of coaching high-level executives in major corporations, but the system can work for anyone. No specialized binders or software are required.

I am personally grateful for his book, because I had always found it impossible to implement a strictly linear prioritized approach to time and task management. From that perspective, another book I've found helpful is *Time Management for Unmanageable People* by Ann McGee-Cooper.

Regardless of the approach you use for conflict resolution and time/task management, these are major areas of personal development. They not only make a person more valuable within a workforce, but also more relaxed and fulfilled. And that's the description of a healthy hedonist at work!

"Your transition between work and home can greatly impact how you feel when you return, and consequently heighten the quality of your evening."

Chapter Twelve

HOME, JAMES!

As a writer, I'm now able to work from home. But after spending more than 25 years working each day at other locations, I have not forgotten the grind. My jobs have been varied, from public relations to turquoise cutting, bookkeeping, and bartending, with some retail and restaurant experience thrown in for good measure.

My turquoise-cutting days were the worst in terms of how I felt at the end of the day. I'd come home cold, wet and dirty, with my fingers cut up and my face caked with dust. I'd been breathing toxic substances all day, and the experience showed me what a day of work is like for those whose jobs expose them to such conditions. Ever since, I've always appreciated the cleanliness of office jobs and being able to come home and place the jacket or sweater I've worn all day back in the closet to wear again.

My early days in public relations were also strenuous, though in a different way. I'd come home brain-dead. All I could handle those evenings was talking on the phone and flipping through catalogs.

Increasingly, though, I had other interests and responsibilities. Besides shopping and cooking, there was also other "work" that needed to be done after I came home. Some of that was energizing, such as my woodworking classes, but some of it became a real chore, such as personal bookkeeping.

My experience has shown me there are things that can be done during the transition time between work and home which will greatly impact how you feel when you return, and consequently heighten the quality of your evening.

HEALTHY SNACKING BEFORE DINNER

One strategy is to *not* arrive home famished. Otherwise, the probability is increased that you will grab whatever you can first put your hands on—healthy or not. Strategic nibbling to keep your blood sugar slightly up also helps ensure that you have enough energy to deal with dinner and the rest of the evening chores.

Apples: For practicality and health, an apple to munch in the car as you're driving home is hard to beat. It's high in fiber, contains no fat and is a tasty way to prevent yourself from getting too hungry, without ruining your appetite for dinner. If you're picking up kids on the way home, having apples for children is one way to help them cope as well. Apples need to be washed before you eat them, so the apples need to be brought from home, or rinsed elsewhere.

Protein bars: I often eat half a protein bar when I'm extremely fatigued. That helps a lot, but I can't say that it doesn't affect my appetite. If I'm just going to go home to eat a light dinner, such as steamed vegetables, it's not a problem. However, I don't recommend eating such a dense food if you have plans to eat a bigger meal.

Soy nuts: I find that soy nuts work well as a dose of protein. This is the kind of thing that I can eat just enough of to prevent hunger pangs and low blood sugar, but not something I find myself losing control with. I personally prefer the honey-flavored ones. They're sold in plastic bags, and I carry them in a pint-sized jar. I find that's the right size to munch from in a moving car. Eating them straight from the bag has not worked too well. The bag often rips, and I end up with soy nuts all over the seat.

Vegetable sticks: The best thing that's happened to carrot sticks is the packaging of prepared baby carrots; you can find these at most grocery stores. The really tiny ones are the sweetest. Even better, you can get organic ones at the health food store. A "celery and nut butter" combo, prepared in the morning, or even the night before, can also work. You can't call that snack low-fat, because of the nut butter. However, this snack provides protein and other nutritional benefits, and it will tame your hunger until dinner.

Juice bar: Some point during the drive home can be a good time to stop by a juice bar for some freshly squeezed juice. This treat can be an excellent and delicious way to survive until dinner. I don't recommend reconstituted, canned or bottled juice. (Read more about this in Chapter 20, "Juicing & Saturday Salads.")

SIMPLE STRESS RELIEF

A yoga class after work, once or twice a week, is a great way to arrive at home feeling very relaxed. I'm a long-term practitioner of yoga and recommend it highly. You'll find it mentioned several times in this book along with a whole chapter on the subject (Chapter 26, "Yoga and T'ai Chi"). Yoga classes, especially from someone with classical yoga training, can be a great way to learn breathing exercises.

If you're not quite ready to learn breathing techniques, consider just taking a moment before you leave the car to sit in silence and blow out tension. Empty your lungs and take a deep breath. As you hold it, say to yourself that when you let go of the breath, you will be relaxed and renewed, ready to spend a lovely evening at home. As you exhale, visualize that you're blowing out all the tension and stress you've accumulated during the day. Do this two or three times if you like. And then smile. It's a worthwhile invest-ment in terms of time.

Another great way to relieve stress is by stopping at a park, a beach or some other place of scenic beauty that isn't too far off the regular route home. This could be a good way to get in a daily walk that will give you not just the exercise of walking, but a larger sense of who you are. To climb to the top of a hill at sunset and then feel a breeze whirl through your hair and blow on your face is guaran-teed to give you a better perspective on the day's events. If you've picked up kids on the way home, this can be an ex-cellent way to allow them to burn off some steam before they arrive home, too.

Another simple way to reduce stress on the way home is to refuse to listen to the news. I understand that you may need to tune into a traffic report or two as you start home, but that doesn't mean you have to leave the news station on. Play your favorite music instead—loud. And sing along! Or whistle. Consider making a personalized tape or CD of songs that, for you, will best help you leave work behind.

Once you arrive home, refuse to become immediately caught up in mail, phone messages, email and dinner prepa-rations. Instead, you might go inside, quickly change into walking clothes, then head straight back out the door for a walk (if you didn't take one earlier). This is another way to rapidly change gears. It's a tip I learned from having dogs, especially dogs who were cooped up in a small house while

I was gone to work. They had a doggie door and could go out back during the day. However, any dog will let you know that being able to get out in the yard during the day is not the same as going for a WALK, WALK, WALK!

A two-minute shower before changing into your comfy evening clothes can rapidly improve your mood. It's my favorite way of shaking off the feel of the road when I've had to drive a long way to go to a meeting. After an especially trying day, you can visualize all the stress and tension going down the drain. This is well worth the time it takes. You'll come out of the bathroom glowing and relaxed, in clean and comfy clothes, and really feel like a different person than the one who came in the door.

"Right-fat, low calorie snacking helps me remain vertical and reasonably pleasant until an actual meal makes it to the table."

Chapter Thirteen

TASTY, RIGHT-FAT SNACKS

A personal habit I've developed is to eat five or six mini-meals a day, rather than just two or three larger ones. I've seen this idea increasingly validated by health research. It's actually not a choice for me. I'm a borderline hypoglycemic, and when my blood sugar gets low, I become irritable and spacey. At such times, there is no higher priority than eating until my blood sugar is back up again. As I have no self-control when faced with this situation, what keeps me from not eating high-fat items is to not have them available in my house in the first place.

Over the years, through experimentation, I've developed strategies for right-fat, low-calorie snacking that help me remain vertical and reasonably pleasant until an actual meal makes it to the table. Experiment with my ideas yourself, and enjoy these healthy snacks.

SMART SNACKING TIPS

My all-time favorite strategy is to heat a *corn tortilla* on the burner of my gas stove. (This doesn't work well on an electric burner. The tortilla will stick to the coils. With an electric stove, you need to heat the tortilla in a little skillet.) After I've flipped the tortilla a couple of times on my gas stove, and its surface is starting to bubble and become browned, I remove the tortilla from the stove. Then I smear it with spicy bean spread.

The great part about this humble snack food is that I can be totally famished, but after eating two of them, three at the very most, I'll be quickly revived. This snack is nutritious and inexpensive, about 17 cents apiece. I can make this treat in under two minutes. It has 80 calories, 2.5 grams of protein, and .75 grams of fat. I usually eat these standing up.

The *bean spread* I buy is sold in little jars, usually displayed near the tortilla chips. If you don't find a similar product at your market, or if you don't like the ones you find, you can easily make something similar yourself. Just mix canned refried pinto beans with salsa—enough of each to end up with a nice flavor and spreading consistency. I recommend the nonfat canned beans to avoid the lard used in the regular products.

Because the beans have been "predigested," so to speak, by the process that turns them into bean spread, they seem to digest much more easily. That is another way to say that I don't notice that they cause flatulence when I eat them. Maybe my stomach has adjusted. If you don't find this to be true for you, my apologies. There are plenty of other ideas to try in this chapter.

THE CHIP EXPERIMENT

One day, I was staring at the rack of tortilla chips at the grocery store, looking hard at the price and thinking about the fat content. I knew I had a large stack of fresh corn tortillas sitting in the refrigerator at home. A moment later, I decided not to buy the commercial chips, but to make my own baked tortilla chips instead.

Fresh corn tortillas make delicious baked chips. I buy them by the 30-count or 50-count stack. You just chop the tortillas into sixths. Arrange the tortilla wedges on a foil-lined cookie sheet. Bake them until they're golden brown in a 450° oven. (You have to keep an eye on them while they're baking. It doesn't take long—maybe seven or eight minutes—and they're done.)

Since I began making chips myself, I'm also happy to report finding a handy, inexpensive microwave chipmaker on the market. (See Resources.) This simple plastic rack allows you to quickly and easily make tortilla, pita or bagel chips. The chips don't tend to burn when cooked in a microwave, so you don't have to watch them. The box warns that you should use a potholder to remove the rack from the microwave.

Whether you make them in the oven or with a microwave rack, home-baked tortilla chips taste significantly different from the conventional tortilla chips you're used to eating. You'll enjoy the light, sweet taste of the corn, without the fat content that comes from the deep-frying process used to make conventional chips. Because they're fresh, your home-baked chips will also have a more delicate flavor than the commercial ones. The homemade ones cost less, and they're a whole lot better for you. If you eat them with salsa, they're a nutritious, right-fat, low-calorie snack. The chips will store well in an airtight container.

WHAT TO DIP YOUR CHIPS IN?

A tip for buying salsa at a lower cost than supermarket prices is to go to a restaurant-supply wholesale grocer. Buy it in a larger container, and break it down into smaller ones.

I was so pleased with the microwave chipmaker that I decided to test other possible kinds of home-made chips, with excellent results. In the chart below, I compare the nutritional content of my homemade chips with commercial chips. The differences in fat content are an eye-opener.

CHIP COMPARISON

Product	Serving Size	Calories Per Serving	Fat Grams Per Serving	Carbohydrate Grams Per Serving	Comments
Commercial tortilla chips	6 chips (1 oz.)	130	6	19	Who stops at six? I can eat a basket of them with margaritas.
Home-baked tortilla chips	6 chips	60	.75	11	Cost less, taste better, more nutritious.
Home-baked pita chips	16 chips (1 pita split, then each half cut in eighths)	70	.25	15	These cook fast in the microwave, taste great and function well as chips. A "steal" in terms of fat and calories.
Commercial potato chips	20 chips (30 gr.)	160	11	14	High fat and habit forming.
Homemade yam chips	40 chips from half a yam	50	.1	11.5	Surprisingly good. They took a little longer to cook, but are worth it.
Commercial fried apple chips	12 chips (1 oz.)	140	7	20	Like other fried chips, high in fat.
Apple slices used as chips	13 thin slices cut from half a small apple	29	.3	7.25	The numbers speak for themselves.

You'll then freeze most of it. Salsa is quite acidic, so it stores well.

Why all this emphasis on salsa? Well, salsa is low in both fat and calories, and it has nutritious ingredients. It's exciting and flavorful enough that you'll feel satisfied by a relatively small amount.

If bean dips or salsas are not to your liking, try *hummus*. It's made from garbanzo beans, lemon juice, tahini (ground sesame seeds) and garlic. Hummus has 70 calories to a two-tablespoon serving, with 40 fat calories and 2 grams of protein.

Babaganooj is much the same as hummus, but it's made from baked eggplant instead of garbanzo beans. It has 25 calories to a two-tablespoon serving, 15 calories from fat, and 1 gram of protein.

These spreads are tremendously satisfying in terms of taste and are very low in fat. You can find either of them in the deli sections of health food stores or supermarkets that carry a large selection of prepared foods. You may also get them at Greek and Middle Eastern restaurants or groceries. I guarantee that you can eat hummus or babaganooj on a rice cake without feeling deprived in the slightest. They are rather garlicky, but hopefully your mate likes garlic too.

"Veggie Pates" are also available at health food stores in a variety of flavors.

MORE SNACKING SUGGESTIONS

A *rice cake with cottage cheese* is still a personal favorite snack, especially with a little seasoning sprinkled on top, such as Spike® or Salt-Free Spike, Vegit® (very low in sodium) or Frontier™ Bombay Veggie Blend. All of these seasonings are available at health food stores. *Pretzels, celery, carrot sticks* and *soy nuts* are reliable standards for snacks. *Vegetarian broths* and lots of *water* are a "secret" way to feel full, suggested at many of the most expensive spas. Home-made vegetable broth is very satisfying and it has lots of minerals to facilitate weight loss and detoxification.

I find that a *hard candy* or two during the day can help a lot when I'm trying to avoid overeating. I keep a small bag of them in my purse and pull them out when I have to drive for an hour or two, or in other tedious situations, like standing in lines.

Baked tofu is a nice right-fat snack. To make it, drain the tofu, cut it in cubes, marinate it in teriyaki or jerk sauce for a half hour or so, then bake it in a 400° oven for 15 to 20 minutes. Jerk sauce is a sweet and spicy Caribbean marinade sauce available in the condiment section of most supermarkets. This might take too much time for a weeknight, but it's a wonderfully nutritious, right-fat and low-calorie *hors d'oeuvre* for parties.

Fresh *fruits* and *veggies* always make great snacks. Grapes are wonderful for nibbling. So are cherry tomatoes, but watch out when you're wearing good clothes. These tomatoes tend to squirt.

Baby carrots are now sold in snack packs, with a small serving of ranch dressing to dip them in. This is probably the best thing that's happened to carrot-nibbling. You can create a similar but healthier combo at home, using low-fat yogurt and a few spices. (See Recipes.) Actually, any kind of veggie can be dipped in this.

I have also seen celery and peanut-butter snack packs at the store, as well as all sorts of flavored veggie dips. Again, you can put something similar together at home.

Here's a combination that you may not have tried. Start

POPCORN VARIATIONS

If you were at all impressed with some of the homemade chip figures in the Chip Chart, *air-popped popcorn* still beats them all if you've really got the *mad munchies*.

Two tablespoons of un-popped corn yields *5 cups(!)* of popped corn which total only 100 calories, 1 gram of fat (0 saturated) and 4 grams of protein.

There are lots of things to do with air-popped popcorn. Pick any one of the following suggestions, and they might inspire you to think of some of your own ideas.

1. Season the popcorn with garlic salt and Parmesan cheese.

2. Lightly toss the popcorn with a teriyaki, ginger and garlic sauce. Such a sauce can be found in the condiments section of most supermarkets.

3. Make a dressing (see Recipes) of olive oil, garlic juice and Bragg's™ Liquid Aminos. If you put this in a spray bottle, you can add it lightly on the popcorn.

4. Try adding nutritional yeast flakes, available from most health food stores, on popcorn. I think it has an interesting taste, and when used on popcorn, it creates a highly nutritious combination. Yeast is high in iron and B vitamins. Popcorn also supplies lots of fiber.

If you have more ideas for air-popped popcorn, email them to me (janet@thehealthyhedonist.com). I'll post your suggestions to our website, *www.thehealthyhedonist.com*.

with jicama, pronounced *hick-a-ma*. It's a grapefruit-sized root vegetable, brown on the outside and white on the inside. It's reminiscent of a potato, but jicama has a sweet crisp flavor, rather similar to an apple. I've never seen it eaten any way but raw. Peel it by slicing off the ends and then pulling off the outside skin. Cut the jicama into half-inch slices. Now squeeze lime juice on it and sprinkle chili powder on that. This is another wonderful party *hors d'oeuvre*. Jicama is a favorite of mine to include on a *crudités* tray (one that offers raw vegetables with a dip).

If you usually have something sweet in mind when you reach for a snack, there are now some wonderful options in the diet or special sections of more upscale supermarkets. These grocery stores provide products for diabetics that taste good and still fit within many dietary recommendations. There are also some healthful options in the cookie sections of health food stores. One variety (Barbara's Oatmeal Cookies) that I tried has reduced fat and is wheat-free and dairy-free. One cookie contained 60 calories, 3 grams of fat (1 saturated) and 8 grams of carbohydrate. It was quite tasty. For persons who are allergic, or otherwise on restricted diets, such products mean you can stay on your program without feeling totally deprived. They can also be good for those of us who are trying to be good most of the time so that we can be really bad occasionally.

Sorbet makes a delicious treat. I find it hard to keep this food on hand. At our house, it always seems to be gone within an hour or two of coming home from the store.

Frozen fruit-juice bars, especially tropical flavors such as coconut and mango, are wonderful in warm weather. I find them almost as satisfying as a cold beer.

I know there are those who will read this section and

have ideas that I haven't discovered. I hope you will accept my sincere invitation to share them with the rest of us at *www.thehealthyhedonist.com.*

GOOD FATS VS. BAD FATS

In his book *Detoxification & Healing: The Key to Optimal Health*, Sidney MacDonald Baker, M.D., devotes an entire chapter, titled "Fat Is Not Just to Hold Your Pants Up," to the role of fats in the composition of our cells and the function of all bodily processes.

Our bodies synthesize fats as a means of storing the energy from sugars and carbohydrates. Yet, in what can only be termed a quirk of nature, our biochemistry is unable to use these stored fats for the production of prostanoid hormones. This type of hormone, which was only discovered in the 1960s, is the short-distance message carrier that enables cells to communicate and therefore harmonize with each other. The body needs to have a supply of two kinds of essential fatty acids to manufacture the prostanoid hormones, which are used *by every cell of the body* for regulating the activity of the cells. The key word here is ESSENTIAL. The fats that are required for this purpose are alpha-linolenic acids, more commonly referred to as omega-3 fatty acids, and linolenic acids, or omega-6 fatty acids.

Omega-3 and omega-6 oils are part of a group of fats called unsaturated fatty acids, because their chemical structure is not "saturated" with hydrogen atoms. Food sources for these oils include corn oil, soybean oil, peanut oil, cottonseed oil, linseed or flaxseed oil, fish oil and marine plant oils. The unsaturated quality of these fatty acids makes them more flexible. Consequently, they are liquid at room temperature, unlike butter, for example. Butter and all other animal fats are saturated fats, as are coconut oil and palm kernel oil.

Another major role of essential fatty acids is for use in building cell membranes. Flexible, unsaturated fatty acids are the body's preferred source for building cell membranes. The body uses whatever oil source it has for this purpose, but does not change the basic composition of the oil it uses. Therefore the oils that you ingest become the actual cell membranes of your body.

Early in the 20th century, food chemists developed hydrogenated oils, or trans-fatty acids (TFAs), as a way of creating an inexpensive butter substitute with a long shelf life. The process forces hydrogen into refined unsaturated oil at high temperature (between 200° and 400° F) in the presence of a metal catalyst, commonly an alloy containing 50 percent nickel and 50 percent aluminum. Not only does the process destroy essential oils, but heavy-metal traces of the catalyst are left in the final product. Hydrogenated oils are now used widely in the making of commercial baked products, fried foods and most chocolates (sad but true!).

Trans-fats interfere with normal biochemistry in many ways. They decrease beneficial HDL cholesterol, interfere with detoxification processes and block the function of essential fatty acids. Dr. Baker makes this easier to understand by saying, "Thick and stiff oils are toxic in that they cause an unwelcome rigidity in cell membranes and do not provide suitable raw materials for making hormones."

Fatty acid deficiencies show up in many ways in the body that you can see. These include:

- Cracking finger tips
- Patchy dullness of the skin, especially on the face

- Mixed oily and dry skin, which is sometimes called *"combination skin"*
- Chicken skin on the back of the arms featuring small, rough bumps
- Alligator skin, usually on the lower legs, which has an irregular quilted appearance with dry patches
- Stiff, dry, unmanageable, brittle hair
- Seborrhea, a type of oily skin
- Cradle cap, a condition seen in infants that features greasy gray or dark scaly crusts on the scalp
- Dandruff
- Hair loss
- Soft fingernails
- Brittle fingernails, which fray with horizontal splitting

Crucial health benefits are derived from the consumption of essential fatty acids. The right intake helps keep blood platelets from sticking together, reduces the possibility of blood clots and contributes to the opening up of blood vessels, improving circulation. If there is a deficiency of essential fatty acids in the diet, as there is in the diets of most Americans, a whole range of circulatory problems including high blood pressure can result. This is directly related to the fact that heart disease is the number one cause of death in the United States.

There is, fortunately, an easy way to improve many of these problems by simply taking a tablespoon a day of flaxseed oil. It's best used to make salad dressings or to add to cooked foods and should never be used for frying, sautéing, or coating pans used for baking. Heat causes flaxseed oil to go rancid. In addition, flaxseed oil must be refrigerated unless it is purchased in flaxseed capsules. It's best to purchase it from a health food store you trust to be sure the product is fresh.

A great deal of research into the omega 3s and 6s continues. Several studies support the premise that alpha-linolenic acid and other omega 3 fatty acids can inhibit cancer formation, may possibly be used for tumor reduction and might even normalize mutated cells. Still other research is attempting to discover the role of essential fatty acids in immune system disorders. My suggestion is not to wait for the research to come in. Increase your supply of omega 3 oil (via flaxseed oil) now.

Besides using flaxseed oil in salad dressings or adding it to a morning smoothie, another way of increasing the amount of flaxseed oil in your diet is to grind organic flaxseeds (surprisingly inexpensive at your health food store) in a coffee grinder and adding them to breakfast cereal or smoothies. I use two tablespoons of the seeds and grind them for about ten seconds. If you don't eat cereal for breakfast, you can stir the ground seeds into a little soy milk, goat's milk, or organic cow's milk to make a mild-tasting paste which is very easy to swallow. The fiber in the ground seeds also makes them very good for keeping your colon clean and healthy. Some people have found the ground flaxseeds to be an extremely effective remedy for constipation. Ground flaxseeds should be used within 45 minutes after grinding the seeds.

In addition to flaxseed oil, olive oil (an omega 6 oil) has been shown to be beneficial by the epidemiological studies that created the phrase "the Mediterranean diet." These studies showed that persons eating a Mediterranean diet not only lived longer, but also had lower rates of coronary heart disease and other chronic conditions including diabetes and cancer. Olive oil withstands heat and is an excellent choice in cooking a wide variety of ethnic cuisines, including Italian, Greek, Chinese, Indian and Thai.

To derive the greatest health benefits, buy a high quality, extra virgin, cold-pressed olive oil.

"Music, whether produced by voice, instrument, or the two in concert, restores our connection with our essence—the realm beyond our conscious awareness—and thus with the cosmos."
Mitchell L. Gaynor, M.D.

"Flowers, music, candlelight and scent create an environment that sounds good, smells good, and looks great, an environment that, very simply, provides pleasure."

Chapter Fourteen

MOOD-ALTERING STRATEGIES

SETTING THE STAGE FOR RELAXATION

There's a point every evening when it's time to wind down. Exactly when that is differs widely from person to person. If you live alone, or with someone whose tastes closely approximate yours, that moment could be as early as when you come in the door. If you have a family, I don't have to tell you that settling down early is usually impossible.

What I'm talking about isn't the stage when you actually change into sleepwear, wash your face, brush your teeth, and turn out the lights. I'm talking about the hour, or hopefully a longer period, when you begin downshifting.

There's a misconception in popular culture. If someone describes a room with fresh flowers on the table, soft music on the sound system, candlelight and perfume in the air, the word "romantic" would immediately pop into your head. You might figure a seduction scene would ensue. I'm not denying the validity of that assumption, but I'd like to expand it. Why can't it be equally true for a person who is spending time alone, or with their mate on an ordinary weeknight?

The hedonistic reason for such indulgence is that the flowers, music, candlelight and scent create an environment that sounds good, smells good, and looks great, an environment that, very simply, provides pleasure. And you deserve such pleasure on a daily basis. You don't have to wait until Saturday night.

Attention male readers! Here's a major hint on how to improve your sex life. If you think you don't care personally for flowers, music, candlelight and nice smells, fake it! Buy flowers anyway. Put on soft music regardless. Go ahead, light the candles. Besides the fact that these small actions will cause you to feel more relaxed, they're even more likely to improve your mate's mood. That's almost guaranteed to make a difference in the bedroom.

From a health perspective, creating such a pleasurable environment can have a tremendous effect in terms of reducing stress, with all the attendant benefits. Pleasure provided this way is low in calories and non-fattening. It fits into any diet strategy and goes a long way toward overcoming feelings of deprivation that you may be experiencing if you're on a restricted diet. This is another kind of soul food. I can breathe in the atmosphere created by the combination of candles, music, aroma and flowers and actually feel physically satisfied by it. Try it yourself and see if it works for you in the same way.

If you live with kids, you may not be able to raise much enthusiasm from them about creating this environment every night. However, they can be gradually taught to appreciate it through a weekly "special family dinner" ritual one night a week. The announcement goes something like "Okay, kids, this is family time. Turn off the tube." With younger kids, it might be a game night or a family video night. Come puberty, it's good to teach them some social graces, along with the art of conversation. Enlist them to help set the table nicely, light the candles and select the dinner music. "Yes, kids, we're going to enjoy each other's company tonight." They might not appreciate the occasions immediately, but learning to sit at a table and eat a civilized meal is excellent preparation for all sorts of adult situations. Also, being a family together around a table forms a circle. The circle is a symbol of familial strength. Research has shown that kids from families that eat together do better in school. It could be because they feel more secure. Or it might be that they learn to participate in adult discussions. Regardless of why it works, when they have grown up and are living in different parts of the country, they will treasure the memory of these occasions.

Even if you can't persuade other family members to forsake the television or the computer most evenings, there is the option of removing yourself to your bedroom to enjoy the benefits of a less stressful environment.

Another room where candles, music and aroma naturally find their place is in the bathroom. (See Chapter 16, "The New Art of Bathing.") A half-hour bath, by candlelight, with music and aromatherapy, is a readily available luxury that most people don't take advantage of. And yet, think what a tiny percentage of people in ancient history had such luxury available to them? To be able to bathe nightly with music, you would have had to be very wealthy to have a bathroom large enough for you and the musicians. Plus, you'd need to be exhibitionistic enough to bathe in front of them. In addition, you would have been considered selfish if you did not share the music with all your family and friends! But now, we've been blessed with the miracle of electronic reproduction that makes music possible and portable at prices everyone can afford.

FLOWER POWER

People have funny notions of cost and extravagance. Huge numbers of folks now think nothing of spending $3 for a latte, $3 for a good loaf of bread and $4 for a box of dry cereal. But flowers, which can last a week and brighten the house to the benefit of all therein, are too frequently thought of as an extravagance—something "only for special occasions."

Here's a cheap and simple experiment. When you go to the market, indulge your senses and your soul by buying one lovely, fragrant rose. Or a bouquet of fragrant carnations. Or whatever type of flower you really love (keeping in mind that this does not have to be an expensive proposition). See what the addition of the flowers does for your week.

Flowers are something that the healthy hedonist buys for himself or herself as a way to bring a sense of luxury into the home on a daily basis. That spot of color draws the eye, catches a corner of your attention and speaks to you with a perky little "hello" that pops into your consciousness as you enter the room.

If you have a home with a garden, planting flowers especially for cutting can be a source of great joy. Many of them grow very easily, such as cosmos, lilies, iris, sweet peas, daisies. There are so many possibilities!

Roses, though a bit more trouble, can provide joy throughout the spring, summer and into fall.

With a bit of planning, you can have flowers in the garden seven or eight months of the year in many climates. In the Sun Belt, you can have them year-round. Though not instantly gratifying, gardening can repay your efforts a hundredfold over time. If you can't imagine finding spare time to tend a whole garden, consider container gardening in large pots or window boxes. It's very Italian, very cheerful. It requires very little energy for the benefit. Ask a helper at a nearby nursery for tips on how to get started or find a book at the library. I've listed one in Resources. This can also be a fun project in which to involve your kids and will teach them some valuable life skills, too.

You can even grow flowers indoors. For instance, you could buy an orchid plant that will give you 30 to 60 days of blossoms for between $18 and $25 at large warehouse home-improvement stores. Even some of the discount retailers have them.

Amaryllis bulbs in fall and winter are another great yet inexpensive treat. It's very sensuous to watch them grow noticeably every day as they shoot that large stem into the air before blooming.

For what is a relatively small amount of money for the pleasure, several catalogs offer flower specials guaranteed to brighten your home during winter. One company offers "4 Months of Spring Color and Fragrance." They send a tabletop planter of blooming spring bulbs each month from December through March. (See Resources.)

THE HEALING EFFECTS OF SOUND

A great deal of research has been conducted in recent years to determine if, and how, music can contribute to healing. Examples of current research include a study by Mark Rider, Ph.D., a research psychologist with Southern Methodist University. Dr. Rider found that music, often combined with imagery, has a powerful positive influence on the protective cells of the immune system. In addition, David Simon, M.D., medical director of neurological services at Sharp Cabrillo Hospital in San Diego and the Chopra Center for Well-Being in La Jolla, California, found that vocal chants are *chemically* metabolized into endogenous opiates with both healing and painkilling effects.

The central principle underlying the healing effects of music, and more broadly, sound, is that of *"entrainment,"* a phenomenon first observed by Christian Huygens in 1665. In the process of making pendulum clocks, Huygens noticed that two pendulums swinging near each other will gradually synchronize. Researchers went on to discover that any two oscillators pulsing at a similar rhythm will gradually synchronize. Additional research found that our bodies, organized around many different rhythms, but especially the rhythm of our heart and lungs, are affected by, and in some cases will actually synchronize with the tempo of different kinds of music or sound.

We understand this instinctively when we dance or fall under the hypnotic effect of a steady drumbeat.

On a cellular level, as well as on the subatomic level of physics, disease can be seen as disharmony. Shamanistic traditions dating back thousands of years have used sound to restore the harmony that is health. New research-based music is being composed and recorded to promote health and harmony with certain powerful sounds, chants, tones and music. (See Resources.)

To relax at home at night, find your own "lullabies," whatever music you enjoy that soothes you and slows you down. Whether it be classical, popular or "world" music is not relevant. This can be facilitated by creating a small library (or libraries in different parts of the house) where you can quickly grab a cassette or CD.

For example, you could stash music to accompany bathing near the bathtub and mood music in the bedroom. One word of caution. Always set any electrical device far enough away from the tub. That way, if something should cause the device to fall, it won't land in the water with you.

SOFT LIGHTING & CANDLES

I've heard some of my most aesthetically gifted friends say, "I hate overhead lighting." Instead of using overhead lighting at home in the evening, they turn on table lighting. Overhead lighting is glaring and unflattering, especially fluorescent lighting. Incandescent bulbs in general provide a softer, warmer light, but even they can be improved upon. I have one friend who goes to the trouble of finding pink lightbulbs to install in her lamps. It's a wonderful way to improve the mood of your home.

It's good "sleep hygiene" to begin turning down the lights a couple of hours before you go to bed. This tells the brain that it will soon be time to go to sleep. Bright lights and sleep are contradictory. You can read more about this in Chapter 18, "Sleep, Blissful Sleep."

Candles are something many people have gotten in the habit of using—with good reason. Candlelight dramatically changes the mood of your home. Candles are mesmerizing for me. I consider them a form of prayer, a reminder of the struggles of someone I love. I love what they do for a table where close friends or family are about to enjoy a meal.

Here is a word of caution about candles: According to the U.S. Consumer Product Safety Commission, 40 percent of candles on the market contain lead wires inside their wicks. These are most often scented candles. The added scent softens the wax and the lead wire is used to make the wick firmer. You can tell that the wick has lead in it if: (1) you peel back some of the cotton wick and can see a metal core; or (2) you rub the tip of the wick across a piece of paper and it leaves a gray pencil-like mark.

Something new on the market is a type of candle made from vegetable source materials, usually corn. You'll probably have to go to a health food store to find these. However, if you're at all chemically sensitive, it's a way of eliminating a source of petrochemicals in your air without giving up the pleasure of candles. If you're sensitive, also look for candles made with essential oils rather than chemical fragrances. You'll learn more about this in the next chapter on aromatherapy.

EVERYDAY PLEASURES

The money and the effort necessary to treat yourself to flowers, music and candles on a regular basis is tiny compared to the pleasure they impart and the degree to which they can reduce your mid-week stress. Don't wait for special occasions. You're special every day of the week!

"Essential oils remind us of the forest and the meadow. They have amazing therapeutic powers, as if it were Mother Nature herself reaching out to soothe and heal us."

Chapter Fifteen

GIFTS OF THE MAGI, GIFTS FOR YOU

You've probably heard the word *"aromatherapy"* used in the marketing of personal care products. But it isn't just a marketing term. This is a serious, research-based body of knowledge on the use of essential oils to promote well-being.

"Essential oils" is the term given to products of distillation that come from pure plant sources. Depending on the plant, that source could be the flowers, leaves, seeds, branches or roots. Typically it is the part that yields the plant's characteristic scent.

Aromatherapy is an enchanting subset of herbal medicine and it serves to remind us of our connection to the natural world—a link that our modern lifestyles tend to obliterate.

Essential oils quite literally "ground" us, but in the lightest and most gentle way. They remind our conscious and unconscious mind of the forest and the meadow, realms where humankind wandered for hundreds of thousands of years before recorded history began. Plus, they have amazing therapeutic powers, as if it were Mother Nature herself reaching out to soothe and heal us. Because the essential oils are powerful and somewhat expensive, it's useful to be consciously aware of what their name implies—essential oils are the "essence" of nature.

Many of the therapeutic effects of essential oils stem from the way scent stimulates the brain's limbic system, where the complex functions of emotion take place. Because an aroma reaches the brain very quickly via the nasal passage, the effect that scent has on the brain is almost instantaneous.

MODERN & ANCIENT USE

Modern therapeutic use of plant-based scents began in France in 1937. Rene-Maurice Gattefosse, a chemist in a perfume factory, accidentally burned himself. Seeking relief, Gattefosse plunged his arm into the nearest vat of liquid. It happened to be lavender essential oil. To his surprise, the burn healed much more rapidly than he expected. He then began to research and document the healing power of plant essences.

Though the term aromatherapy is modern, the art and science behind it are not. As long ago as 6,000 years, in the Fertile Crescent of Mesopotamia and Babylon, humans began using scent. Ancient Egyptians became proficient at the art and Cleopatra reputedly soaked her sails in jasmine oil in her efforts to attract Mark Antony. The Bible's nativity story recounts how three wise men honored the infant Jesus with gifts of gold, frankincense (which was then used as incense in its natural state as a tree gum resin) and myrrh (another gum resin often used to make incense). We now have frankincense essential oil.

At one time, the art and science of using scent to affect emotions was considered sufficiently powerful to be banned as sorcery!

Despite the mystique, essential oils are easy to use and they are undoubtedly one of the most luxurious forms of stress management available. If you're looking for a way to lighten your load, this could be it. Aromatherapy is extremely convenient. A bottle of essential oil is tiny; you can easily carry it with you to work or while traveling.

One warning about essential oils is that they're usually not for internal use (only a few are used as flavorings and in very small quantities). Also, because they're strong, essential oils should not be applied directly, full strength, to the skin. They can be diluted in a "carrier oil" such as almond, apricot or sesame oil and then applied on the skin. Some people are allergic to particular oils. If you think you might be allergic, test one oil at a time by applying a diluted drop to a spot on your skin and watching for a reaction. If you're pregnant, consult a qualified aromatherapy specialist before using the oils.

A number of products have been developed to make using essential oils very easy. Among them are ceramic rings that rest on top of a light bulb and "lamps" that use a votive candle to warm a small dish. For both of these, you would mix a small amount of water with a few drops of an essential oil. The heat from the flame gradually evaporates the water, releasing the oil into the air.

There are also necklaces or ornaments to hang in your car. Both hold a small amount of diluted oils. Either one can help you decompress from work.

When added to a carrier oil, most essential oils can be used for skin moisturizing. Only a few will be drying on the skin. (Those include citrus or cedarwood oil.) The rest of the oils can be used in a moisturizing skin oil you can make for yourself. Simply purchase a small quantity (eight ounces

6 WAYS TO USE THESE ESSENTIALLY WONDERFUL OILS

1. Add a few drops to bath water.
2. Shake a couple of drops on a tissue, handkerchief or cotton ball, then stash it in your pocket or under the seat of your car—wherever you'll be able to smell the fragrance over a period of time.
3. Put a few drops into water in a spray bottle. Now spray the air, your sheets or anything else that strikes your fancy.
4. Use that same spray bottle when you're ironing. You could spray the ironing board first, but also use the scented water to dampen wrinkles. This will make ironing much more pleasant.
5. Sprinkle a few drops of a less expensive oil, such as a citrus, into your mop water when cleaning the floor. Magically, you'll clean your psyche without breathing toxic chemicals.
6. Soothing and relaxing aromatherapy combinations using chamomile, lavender and marjoram can be added to bath water to help settle children down before bed. Children love the mystery and beauty of different scents. One more word of caution: Essential oils are not appropriate for children to play with unsupervised. They should be stored well away from your children's reach, as you would any medication.

or less) of a high-quality carrier oil at the health food store. Add a few drops of your favorite essential oil. *Voila!* It's that easy! You can also make a custom blend of oils and develop a "signature" scent. If you find a scent that you particularly like, you can add it to any fragrance-free shampoos available at health food stores. There are books on perfume making listed in Resources that can give you ideas on how to start.

If you're ready for experimentation, there are also books that provide easy recipes for all sorts of personal care products—all made with natural ingredients and essential oils. Trying these recipes can be a fun and creative experience. This is a good foul weather activity, something that works well with family, friends or all by yourself. It's also a way to create unique and affordable holiday gifts.

As you'll see from the chart on the last page of this chapter, different scents carry different emotional connotations and have very different uses. Citrus oils are lively and energizing. Pine is refreshing. Geranium is balancing. Peppermint is stimulating. Lavender is calming. Ginger is warming. Ylang-ylang is often recommended for its sensuality. Frankincense is said to ease the pain of mourning.

We're already familiar with many of these scents because some approximation of them has been used in commercial products of all kinds. Eucalyptus is one we know through numerous products for colds and respiratory conditions. With others, such as cinnamon and pine, we have natural associations from our lives. Even an occasional use of aromatherapy gives one the experience of how a scent evokes images, feelings and memories. And as you use them, the scents will create new associations.

Some oils are strictly therapeutic. For example, tea tree

oil has a strong medicinal smell and it's very effective in first aid. It's anti-bacterial, anti-viral, anti-fungal and anti-septic. But I doubt you'd want to use it in your bathwater to relax.

Blends can be made to use for multiple purposes. For instance, an oil for rubbing into sore joints or muscles is made with four drops each of lavender, birch, cypress and juniper oils. Add these four essences to a carrier oil such as almond or sesame. This is also a stress-reducing combina-tion that can be blended into bathwater or used in a diffuser or other aroma delivery system.

If you're not quite ready to mix and match your own combinations, you can conveniently indulge in all the ben-efits of aromatherapy by simply stopping by a health food store in your area and selecting a blend of oils or a wide assortment of personal care products off the shelf.

INDULGE YOUR SENSES AT THE HEALTH FOOD STORE

There has been an explosion of creativity and product development in personal care products made with natural ingredients and essential oils. Many of the companies (see Resources) have coordinated product lines. They offer, for example, lavender shampoo, conditioner, bath gel, bath salts and skin moisturizer. The packaging is beautiful; the scents are a delight. Besides lavender, other coordinated scented lines use rosemary and mint, lemon verbena, vanilla or rose with chamomile.

You may not have heard the names of the companies that make these products, but that's good. It tells you that you're paying for quality ingredients, not the product's ad-vertising and packaging. Are they expensive? Like any quality product, they're more expensive than the cheap stuff you might buy at a discount store. But they're not at all expensive when you consider the legitimate therapeutic benefits you can derive from using them. These are products that are truly a "plus" for your health, because:

1. They use real essential oils.
2. They're made from natural ingredients. Most of the personal care products on the marketplace are made from petrochemicals that are absorbed through the skin into your bloodstream. They then become something else for your liver to detoxify. Essential oils, by contrast, place no such burden on your system.

ON FRAGRANCES & PERFUMES

Understanding essential oils also teaches us something very important about fragrances and perfumes. All perfumes used to be made of essential oils. That's why they were expensive, something only wealthy people could afford. Since the middle of the 20th century, almost all fragrances are chemically derived. Originally, perfume chemists developed chemical combinations that mimicked the scent of natural substances. Then they created chemical fragrances that were scents unto themselves.

The truth about these chemically-based scents is little known. If I had not personally witnessed the experiences of people who had become chemically sensitive, I might not have believed it. However, we know that chemically-based scents are neurotoxins—that is, they are toxic to the nervous system. If a person is chemically sensitive, just a whiff can cause an instant headache, nausea and other flu-like symptoms that may last for days. So as not to unwittingly affect someone, use *"aroma etiquette."* That is, go lightly with the scents, or forego them entirely, when you are going to be in public or using public transportation, including airplanes. Chemical sensitivity is a growing problem. Awareness is becoming more widespread. I now see meeting notices or signs in doctors' offices that specify "Please, don't wear fragrance." As awareness grows, scents will become something we use in private, not in public.

As you become more aware, you can test your own sensitivity. Does your nose tickle when you walk down the detergent aisle at the supermarket or when you receive a magazine or bill insert advertising perfume? If so, you're reacting to the chemicals.

NOTES FOR COLLECTING THE OILS

Knowing the difference between chemically based scents and those made with essential oils will give you a lot more respect for essential oils. Some are relatively rare. On average, it takes 4,000 kilograms of rose petals (*Rosa damascena*) to produce 1 kilogram of rose essential oil. Producing this oil also requires the labor of many hands to gather and distill the petals. Other oils such as lavender, pine and citrus are relatively inexpensive.

As you gradually begin to accumulate a personal aromatherapy collection, cost will be a factor. You will want to buy from a reputable supplier (see Resources) so that you know you're receiving good value. Comparing the different costs of essential oils is a quick way to judge whether you're buying from an honest company. If the oils are all priced the same, there's a problem. Pine or lemon oil should not cost the same as rose, frankincense or ylang-ylang. Look for a company that's well established, with good connections with its suppliers.

You can find quality essential oils and diffusers in most of the large health food stores. You'll find names of quality Internet-based vendors in the Resources section in the back of this book.

Enjoy the pleasing scents of these wonderful oils!

ESSENTIAL OILS

	balancing	refreshing	cleansing	calming	energizing	use	description	cost	safety
chamomile *Anthemis nobilis*				X		stress reduction, sleep-inducing	replenishing	QE	
cinnamon *Cinnamomum zeylanicum*		X				chills	fresh, spicy, warming	M	SKIN
clary sage *Salvia sclarea*	X					depression, muscle cramps, PMS, stress reduction	warm & woody	M	PG
cypress *Cypressus sempervirens*	X	X	X			fatigue	pine-like	M	
eucalyptus *Eucalyptus globulus*			X		X	colds, asthma, bronchitis headaches PMS antiseptic	familiar through use in cold-related products.	L	
frankincense *Boswellia thurifera*						grief, severe stress, insomnia	sweet balsamic, lemony, peppery	QE	
geranium *Pelargonium graveolens*	X					stress-reducing roselike	powerful	M	PG
ginger *Zingibur officinale*				X		nausea & indigestion, chills	warm	M	
grapefruit *Citrus paradisi*	X	X				depression, PMS	cheering	L	SUN
jasmine *Jasminum grandiflorum*				X		depression, memory problems	sensual, exotic	VE	
juniper *Juniperus communis*					X	acne, eczema, arthritis & rheumatism	woody, fruity, pine-needle scent, good on detox days	M	PG
lavender *Lavendula officinalis*	X			X		insect bites, stress reduction	elegant, called universal calming oil	L	

ESSENTIAL OILS (Cont.)

	balancing	refreshing	cleansing	calming	energizing	use	description	cost	safety
marjoram *Marjorana*				x		antispasmodic, muscular aches & pains	peppery, herbaceous	M	PG
myrrh *Commiphora myrrha*	x					ancient perfume incense component	meditative, a complex balsamic scent	QE	
orange *Citrus sinensis*		x			x	good for "wake up" baths.	bright and cheerful	L	SUN
peppermint *Mentha piperita*		x			x	digestive disorders fatigue, irritable bowel sydrome, headaches & sinus	cooling, deters insects	M	SKIN-PG
pine *Pinus species*		x			x	fatigue	familiar through use in household products	L	SKIN
rose *Rose damascena*						anxiety, PMS	romantic and sensual	VE	PG
sandalwood *Santalum album*	x			x		depression, insomnia stress reduction	rare, sensual	VE	
tea tree oil *Melaleuca alternifolia*						antiseptic, antifungal effective for cuts, bruises, burns, stings, pimples, muscle aches, sores	strong medical odor, immune system stimulant	M	SKIN
ylang ylang *Cananga odorata*	x			x		confidence-building	exotic, sensual	M	

Price Code: L = Low
M = Moderate
QE = Quite Expensive
VE = Very Expensive

Safety Code: SKIN = Dilute well, skin irritant.
SUN = Avoid use in the sun.
PG = Avoid if pregnant.

"Beauty sat bathing by a spring,
Where fairest shades did hide her;
The winds blew calm, the birds did sing,
The cool streams ran beside her."

Anthony Munday

"Bathing is not only available and convenient, it's also affordable. Anyone who complains of not having time for a bath is fooling themselves about whose fault that is."

Chapter Sixteen

THE NEW ART OF BATHING

Note to male readers: I know bathing is something women do far more often than men, but don't skip this chapter. I guarantee that you'll learn something. And sometime in the future, if you've had a disappointing day, you're coming down with a cold or you just feel bored with what's on TV—try taking a bath. The men I know who bathe most often are very masculine. One is a wonderful mechanic who finds it's the best way to get clean after a day in the shop and the other is a kick-ass drummer who really loves the way it helps him relax. What's not to like? This is one of the most hedonistic pleasures in life!

AN ODE TO OUR SMALLEST ROOM

First, allow me a few words of praise for bathrooms. With all the problems our post-modern world presents, there are also achievements worthy of unanimous praise. In this case, I honor our well-plumbed bathrooms. Plus, these rooms come equipped with a door—one that people generally respect. Go in, close the door, and for at least a half hour, most family members won't interrupt you.

Result? A place of sanctuary exists in the bathroom that makes it possible for each of us to "get away from it all" on a regular basis—without spending money we may not have, without sparking "abandonment" issues among family members and without raising questions of paid versus unpaid leave with bosses.

Though the bathroom is the smallest room of the house, it has a large capacity. It is not just for cleaning oneself externally, but also for rejuvenation, relaxation and internal detoxification. It can also enhance your self-esteem—through the simple process of taking time to be good to yourself.

WHY BATHING?

This goldmine of self-care is not only available and convenient, it's also affordable. Anyone who complains of not having time for a bath is fooling themselves about whose fault that is.

What do you think are the short-term benefits of *not* taking care of yourself? Well, in the long run, they're going to cost you BIG TIME in terms of health. And then, how are you going to be able to enjoy life? So take time for yourself, for your health's sake and for the sake of the people who love and depend on you.

Let's look at a simple cost/benefit ratio on bathing.

Two or three nice baths per week require no more than an hour and a half.

They accomplish:

- *Cleaning and grooming of your body.* You were going to spend this time in the bathroom anyway for these purposes.
- *Relaxation.* Collapsing and relaxing aren't the same thing, though collapsing can take up the time that might have been spent in healthier relaxing.
- *Stress reduction.* Here's where the bonus points re-

ally start to accumulate. Time spent in this category will create huge benefits in other parts of your life in terms of greater joy, less irritability, greater ability to cope with whatever your job or life hands you and better health. This will also lead to more energy, more flexibility in your neck and shoulders, less pain in the small of your back, clearer thinking, more resilience and better immune system response. This list could go on and on.

- *Internal tissue detoxification.* What I refer to as "detox" bathing is a gentle process that helps neutralize biochemical imbalances in your body. If you go at it gradually, you won't be aware, initially, that anything is happening. You'll just feel clean and relaxed, as you expect to feel after a bath. Over a period of weeks, the process, combined with other healthy hedonist activities, should give you more energy. Fatigue is the primary symptom of toxicity. Detox bathing can help to reverse it.
- *Pleasure.* Finally. The intrinsic reward.

The bathroom's small area emphasizes the intimate nature of bathing. One sees photos of large bath rooms in glossy decorating magazines, but I don't care for a feeling of openness while I bathe—I'll leave that feeling for when I go to the beach or a swimming pool. I prefer a small bathroom that becomes steamy and warm, and allows me to feel safe and secure. (More later about how to use your own bathroom as a steam room in Chapter 28, "Spa Culture without Big Bucks.")

As we ease into hot, bubbly water, tension sloughs off. A profound experience takes place. It is the return to the liquid environment we experienced both *in utero* and in the deep recesses of our evolutionary past.

A LITTLE HISTORY

Imagine the delight it must have brought our ancestors to find a safe swimming hole on a summer's day. A hot spring would have been even rarer. In Roman times, bathing bubbled up, so to speak. There were 856 public baths in Rome at the end of the 4th century, and the Romans built baths in all the lands they conquered. They used water and bathing therapeutically, as well as for cleansing and social rituals.

With the fall of Rome, bathing lost its social status. After a long hiatus, interest in classical antiquity reemerged in 18th century Europe and brought renewed interested in bathing. By the early 19th century, it had become fashionable to travel to spas and "take the waters." The English city of Bath was named for its baths, as was the German city of Weisbaden, a name that translates as "meadow bath."

Though the Victorians initially considered it indulgent to devote an entire room to bathing, a bathroom soon became a status symbol, and with it, the luxury of the bath returned.

Other cultures have had far more enlightened approaches to bathing for a very long time. The Japanese tradition of "*ofuros*," very hot public baths is just one of these.

Gratefully, our society today accepts bathing as recreation. Swimming pools, hot tubs and backyard spas are not unusual. Bathtubs that incorporate water jets for a whirlpool effect are available and affordable. Even less expensive are bubble massage mats.

In general, the accessories we use today for bathing are

wonderful and inexpensive—cushions for the back and shoulders, little racks to prop up a book, brushes and mitts of all kinds. These are very inexpensive indulgences.

DETOX BATHING

The bath can be a way to gently, effectively and affordably detoxify. How can you tell if you need to detox? The simplest answer is that unless you're living on a mountain top and consuming nothing but organic foods and purified water, you can assume you do. Though we're not exposed to what are considered "deadly" chemical levels, we're ingesting chemicals daily in small amounts from the air, food and water, as well as through our personal habits. Regularly taking antioxidant vitamins, eating lots of fresh fruits and vegetables, getting exercise and all the other behaviors that are usually considered healthy—those activities all play a role in helping your body eliminate toxins. If you're not doing those things, the toxins are accumulating and you could be feeling the results in the form of fatigue. Even more serious illness can result.

Some people have far greater exposure to toxins than others. For example, if you're around smoke, exhaust or chemicals while you're working, or if your job requires you to use protective clothing because of chemical exposure, you might consider finding a less toxic work environment. Otherwise, severe or deadly illness may result.

See our affiliated website, *www.detox.org*, for a more complete description of sources of toxicity and what to do about them.

Here's something easy to do to gently reduce toxins: Several ingredients or techniques can be used in "detox bathing." Try them all, then rotate, as the effect of all but Epsom salts will diminish over time.

It's important to remember that detoxification is a powerful technique that should be approached with respect. If you're ill, weak, pregnant, have high blood pressure or know that you've been exposed to high levels of pesticides, fumigants or industrial chemicals, it is advised to consult your physician before initiating a personal detox program. Or you could seek out a *licensed* holistic practitioner who is familiar with detoxification procedures.

Use common sense. If you're not in the regular habit of bathing, start with only five minutes and work up to a half hour. If at any time you begin to feel faint or nauseous, remain seated in the tub, drain the water and let the feeling subside. Wait until you can climb out safely.

How does detoxification in the bath work? First, let me reassure you that it's a natural process. All you're doing is helping it to happen. According to Drs. Bennett and Barrie in the *7-Day Detox Miracle*, the heat of the warm water causes blood to circulate more quickly. Perspiration begins. Toxins stored in fat cells are naturally excreted as an element of the bodily fluids that are "sacrificed" to perspiration. See the boxed instructions on how to enjoy your own detox bath.

A DETOX BATH HOW-TO

1. Drink a glass of filtered or distilled water before, during and after your bath. Take antioxidant vitamins, as described in the next chapter (Chapter 17, "A Time of Peace"), plus an extra dose of Vitamin C before your bath. These are the biochemical "escorts" required to facilitate detoxification. (More on this in Chapter 25, "Detox Weekends.")

2. Clean the tub with a nontoxic cleanser such as baking soda, Bon Ami® or just clean rags. The logic should be apparent. It makes no sense to clean the bathroom with toxic chemicals, which you inhale while cleaning, immediately before your detox bath!

3. Start by showering and scrubbing yourself down with a loofa sponge, sisal mitt or a rough washcloth to exfoliate dead skin cells. Meanwhile, the hot water and steam will begin to open your pores.

4. Rinse the tub, then fill it as high as possible with water that's as hot as you can tolerate. Block the overflow valve to get the water a little higher. Soak as long as you're comfortable.

5. After soaking, take another shower using soap made from vegetable ingredients and essential

oils. Many delightful handmade soaps of this kind are available at health food stores, farmers markets and natural products boutiques.

6.   Wash your hair and dry it with a clean towel.

Over a couple of weeks, increase the time you stay in the bath to 30 minutes. Once you've acclimated yourself to a half-hour soak, you can add one of the following substances to the bath. (Not all of them at the same time, choose just one.)

- *Epsom salts*—Start by using 1/4 cup of Epsom salts and gradually increase up to four cups per tub. I recently bought a box for $2.49 and this was enough for at least two baths, using the maximum amount. The salts increase perspiration by causing more blood to be supplied to the skin.

- *Apple cider vinegar*—Start off with 1/4 cup, and gradually increase to 1 cup per tub. The vinegar also increases perspiration. Use only apple cider vinegar.

- *Hydrogen peroxide*—When added to the bath, hydrogen peroxide increases the level of oxygen in the blood feeding the cells. It gives you a greater feeling of alertness, which is good, unless you're trying to go to sleep. Try this method when you're preparing to go out for the evening: Buy three bottles of 3% hydrogen peroxide. Fill the tub with warm (not hot) water. (The active ingredient deteriorates rapidly in very hot water.) First add one bottle. Then add a half a teaspoon of sea salt. After five minutes, if no irritation is experienced, add a second bottle. And again, after another five minutes without irritation, add the third. Relax and enjoy the bath for 15 to 20 minutes.

• *Baking soda*—Eight ounces of baking soda, added to the bath, will improve the acid/alkaline balance of your body via osmosis. A body PH that is more alkaline is the result of a healthy diet of fruits and vegetables and less meat, dairy and prepared foods. This is a very easy way to help achieve that balance.

A bathing detox process can be done as often as three times a week while you're working to actively reduce your body's toxicity. You'll know when you're succeeding by your energy level. When you begin to have more energy, as well as a greater sense of mental clarity and "lightness," you've succeeded in reducing your level of toxicity. After that, once or twice a week is a good maintenance frequency.

See footnote at the end of this chapter.

HERBAL BODY TEAS

There are a number of herbs, commonly used as teas, which assist the detoxification process by promoting perspiration. In each case, brew a cup of tea and add it to the bath. Maybe make two cups, one to drink and one to bathe in.

Alphabetically, these herbs are:

- blessed thistle (*Cerbenia* benedicta)
- boneset (*Eupatorium perfoliatum*)
- catnip (*Nepeta cataria*)
- chamomile (*Matricaria chamomilla*)
- horsetail (*Equisetum arvense*)
- peppermint (*Mentha piperita*) and
- yarrow (*Achillea millefolium*).

A good health food store will sell most of these. Peppermint and chamomile can be found in any supermarket's tea section.

These are some other helpful herbs:

- *Lavender* is a superb herb to add to a bath. It's not only calming, but smells wonderful, too. Like other herbs, it promotes perspiration.

- *Gingerroot* improves circulation and draws toxins to the surface of the skin. Make a ginger tea with a two-inch piece of ginger, cut into pieces. Allow it to steep for a half hour and then add the tea to the bath water. Gingerroot can be purchased in the produce section of most groceries and costs only pennies. Ginger is a warming spice, so this is a great herb to use in the wintertime. In addition, add ginger to the bath anytime you've got chills that make you think you're coming down with a bug.

- *Oatstraw* aids detoxification by improving skin metabolism. Simmer a handful in two quarts of water for about a half hour, strain, then pour the oatstraw tea into a tubful of bath water. Oatstraw can be found in health food stores and herbal shops.

A HERBAL BEDTIME TREAT

Detox bathing can be a luxurious way to begin improving your health, and here's a way to stretch that feeling even further. Think of this the next time you change your bedding. Add a couple of drops of lavender essential oil—the universal calming oil—to water in a spray bottle, then spray the clean sheets lightly.

That night, take a nice long bath, put on clean pajamas, crawl between the fresh sheets and enjoy the lovely scent. Ahhhhhhhhh!

* If you implement a combination of healthy hedonistic activities and don't start to feel more energy within a couple of weeks, it would be good to check with your physician or a licensed holistically oriented practitioner who is familiar with detoxification procedures to determine what is causing your fatigue.

"There's a point in the evening when it's time to settle and soothe yourself and meet your own needs for repose."

Chapter Seventeen

A Time of Peace

It's late. You're bone tired. You've made it through the day and are just about ready to crawl into bed.

Does enough sleep await so that you'll wake up in the morning with the energy and enthusiasm to tackle tomorrow's tasks? Or will you lie awake, tossing and turning, occasionally glancing at the slow-moving clock?

Sleep disorders are complex and relate to numerous hormonal, biochemical and emotional issues that vary according to an individual's health, age, sex, diet, stressors and behaviors. It's not possible in this chapter and the next to give you more than a brief overview of how to improve your sleep. If you find that you need more information, consult the Resources section.

However, there are a number of small things which, when done consistently, can help insure a good night's sleep. The last three chapters have presented some of them. As I hope you've noticed, the purpose of these activities is to establish a point in the evening when it's time to settle and soothe yourself and meet your own needs for repose.

If you've previously used the time right before sleeping for journal writing, stretching or meditation, you're on the right track.

HEALTHY HEDONISTS TAKE THEIR VITAMINS

I mention vitamins and other nutritional supplements in this chapter of the book because I take most of my vitamins with dinner because they are best absorbed with a meal. If I forget, I take them right before I go to bed.

However, if you have trouble digesting supplements, the time right before sleeping would not be right for you. Supplements will digest more easily if you take them in the morning with food. Take all of them with breakfast except calcium, which should be taken before bed because it promotes sleep.

There seems to be a fair amount of agreement on the supplements that facilitate detoxification, and I recommend them highly. The list I'm offering in this chapter is derived from numerous sources, including *The 20-Day Rejuvenation Diet Program* by Jeffrey Bland, Ph.D., *Natural Liver Therapy* by Christopher Hobbs, L.Ac., *The Detox Diet* by Elson M. Haas, M.D. and *Prescription for Nutritional Healing* by James F. Balch, M.D., and Phyllis A. Balch, C.N.C.

The authors do not exactly agree on quantities. I've listed conservative amounts. What's important to know is that vitamins and nutrients need to be taken in balanced quantities. Although I know many people who only take one or two of these, there's a payoff in terms of better health from the combination. If you're going to cut corners, this is definitely not the corner to cut.

If you've never taken supplements before, you might have trouble digesting them initially. I'd recommend ramping up with one of the "all-in-one" products mentioned in Recommendations so your system has a chance to adjust.

I firmly believe that taking supplements is one of the most important things to do for your health on a daily basis. Why? Well, unless you're eating lots of farm-fresh produce, you won't absorb sufficient vitamins and minerals from your food, in the proper ratio, to foster the detoxification processes that are essential to your well-being.

To more fully understand why supplements are so important, I suggest you read *Detoxification & Healing: The Key to Optimal Health*, by Sidney MacDonald Baker, M.D. In the meantime, read the expanded explanation of "How the Body Detoxifies" on our affiliated website, *www.detox.org*.

SUPPLEMENTS—A LIST FOR DAILY USE

The following list includes the vitamins and nutrients to be taken daily, along with the appropriate amounts.

Vitamins

Vitamin C (buffered or Ester-C), 500-2,000 mg.

Vitamin E (tocopheryl acetate), 200-400 I.U.

Vitamin A, 5,000-7,500 I.U.

Beta Carotene, 15,000-30,000 I.U.

Bioflavonoids, 200-1,000 mg. (Possibly in a product that combines these with Vitamin C)

B Vitamins (probably in a B compound tablet)

Thiamine (B1), 10-25 mg.

Riboflavin (B2), 10-25 mg.

Niacinamide (B3), 50 mg.

Niacin (B3), 50-2,000 mg.

Pantothenic acid (B5), 250-500 mg.

Pyridoxine (B6), 10-25 mg.

Cobalamin (B12), 50-100 mcg.

Choline (B Family), 500 mg.

Biotin (B Family), 200-300 mcg.
Folic acid (B Family), 400-800 mcg.

Minerals (probably in a mineral tablet or solution)
Zinc (picolinate or oxide), 10-30 mg.
Magnesium, 500 mg.
Manganese (gluconate), 5-10 mg.
Copper (gluconate), 1-3 mg.
Potassium, 50-500 mg.
Molybdenum (sodium molybdate), 50-200 mcg.
Selenium, 50-200 mcg.

Amino Acids (probably in a general blend; 500-1,000 mg. total)
L-cysteine, 100-300 mg.
L-glutathione, 50-200 mg.
L-methionine, 250-500 mg.

Herbs
Note: The following are optional, but can provide important additional support. Follow the recommendations suggested on the packaging.
Garlic (fresh garlic also contains valuable enzymes)
Silymarin (milk thistle)
Pycnogenol
Ginkgo biloba

Women should add a calcium supplement (1000 mg.). This is not only extremely important for preventing osteoporosis, but also helps to induce sleep. Calcium citrate is the form of calcium most easily absorbed by the body. Choose a supplement that combines calcium and magnesium.

MORE SUPPLEMENT TIPS

A good health food store will be able to help you select products that provide these nutrients in the least number of capsules. There are protein powder products that combine all the supplements at the recommended levels. Beyond the protein powders, you probably will not be able to find all the supplements at optimal levels in a single product.

If you have problems with vitamins upsetting your stomach, work with the vitamin specialist at your health food store to find products that are easier to digest. It could be that you would do better with one of the protein powders mentioned above that includes most of them. You may also be able to find some of the supplements in liquid form or in an easily assimilated powder such as Vitamin C powder.

How you take vitamins can make a huge difference in their digestibility. If you make a morning smoothie, adding liquid or powdered vitamins can be an easy way to take them.

If you don't have any luck finding workable solutions with the health food store personnel, it's worth consulting with a nutritionist on this issue. Long-term, nutritional supplementation can make a tremendous difference to your health, so figuring out how to make it work for you is important.

A FEW BEDTIME STRETCHES

It's time to say good night but your stiff muscles won't let you sleep. Painkillers or muscle relaxants may mask the symptoms but they're just another chemical for your liver to detoxify. What can you do? Well, yoga can help release the tension in the muscles and it encourages the lymph and circulation systems to carry off toxins. Thus, you're assisting your body's detoxification processes, rather than giving them an additional load. If you've never tried it, know that yoga works wherever you are. It's not competitive, not even with yourself. It's a welcoming technique that teaches a gentle way to temporarily shelve the pressures of your life and spend a little time taking care of you.

In just a couple of minutes, you can do the following exercises that will help to allow a feeling of calm to settle into your body. These are all poses that are very simple to achieve, whether you've ever done yoga before or not.

STANDING FORWARD BEND

This pose was presented in greater detail in Chapter 11, "Work in Balance."

1. Begin with your feet hip-width apart.

2. Raise your hands over your head and inhale.

3. As you exhale, bend forward from the hips. Your hips should form the corner of the angle. Keep your arms stretched out as you move downward.

4. Continue to bend over as far as you can without straining in any way.

5. Now grab your elbows, relax your shoulders and concentrate on breathing.

That's all there is to it. Close your eyes and just hang and breathe big deep breaths. First you'll feel it in the back of your thighs. That's good. But you should gradually feel your back relaxing. Let your neck loosen.

6. After about a minute, finish by first extending your arms. Next, stretch them out in front of you and straighten up, making a wide arch with your hands. Inhale as you come back up to a standing position with your arms overhead.

EASY BACK STRETCH

1. Sitting cross-legged, stretch your arms overhead.
2. Gradually bend forward, bending from the hips and exhaling as you bend.
3. When you've gone as far forward as you easily can, allow your arms to fall naturally onto the floor in front of you. Allow your arms, neck and shoulders to go completely limp.

Don't struggle with the pose, just breathe. With each breath, you'll feel yourself move an itsy-bitsy, tiny bit further toward the floor. Even if the movement is not visible to the eye, your body feels it. You want the movement to be in your hips and the small of your back (that spot where you accumulate so much stress). If I begin to experience low back pain, I know it's time to get down on the floor and do some stretches. Again, you're using your breath and the weight of your body to work it out.

CHILD'S POSE

After a minute or so of breathing into the previous position, inhale and sit back up. Now switch to kneeling and sit on your haunches.

1. As you slowly exhale, gradually lean forward.
2. Place the top of your forehead onto the floor. As you do this, allow your arms to go backward toward your feet.
3. Then go limp. Just relax and breathe.

This is called the Child's Pose, and it is one of the most simple yet comforting of all yoga positions. In it, you're achieving something close to a fetal position on the floor. It works on a deep psychological and neurological level. But the pose also gives a nice gentle stretch to the back. It's a reassuring pose. You'll find it's an easy position to stay in. Take deeper and deeper breaths and let the tension go.

SPINAL TWIST

We accumulate a lot of stiffness in our neck, shoulders and back from sitting at a desk or driving a car. Perhaps you've noticed that it isn't as easy as it used to be for you to look back over your shoulder when you need to change lanes. Spinal twist is the perfect pose to help that. And being able to check your blind spot before changing lanes is so critical to your safety that I shouldn't have to elaborate too much on why you might want to help yourself to be able to do it quickly and with ease.

The spinal twist is a bit complex. It's a movement in which it's important to remember NEVER to pull or strain, but to relax and breathe into the pose. Be very gentle with yourself on this one.

1. Sit on the floor with your legs extended.
2. Bend the left leg and cross it over the right knee.
3. With your left arm supporting you behind your buttock, raise your right arm and gently turn to the left. Keeping the right arm straight, lower it to the left side of your knee. With this, you have a lever to twist to the left.
4. Turn your torso gently to the left to the furthest point that it will go, then gradually continue to twist to the left with your shoulders and finally with your chin.
5. When you get to the point that's the furthest you can go without straining, just breathe into the pose for at least 30 seconds.

In addition to restoring suppleness to your back, shoulders and neck, visualize that your body is wringing toxins out of your kidneys and adrenal glands. Release and repeat the pose in the other direction.

If you feel too stiff to do this, you can do the modified version, which is performed sitting in a chair. You'll find it in Chapter 11, "Work in Balance."

CREATIVE, PRODUCTIVE WORRYING

Before bed is not the time to worry. But by talking about it here, you're more likely to understand why you need to find another slot every day, or maybe a couple of times each week, to do some highly creative and productive worrying. That way, you won't do it as you lie in bed, trying to fall asleep.

You might need a little notebook for your creative worrying. Or you might create files in your laptop. You could use a page in your organizer or journal. This needs to be something you carry around with you. The next time you find yourself worrying about something, pull out that notebook or open a computer file in the laptop and write down what you find yourself worrying about. At least a couple of times a week, you're going to sit down and focus on exactly what you're going to do to resolve that concern. You're going to plan action steps, prioritize the activities and begin to implement them. You may need to schedule appointments to talk with your mate, boss, neighbor or relative. But then, when that worry comes up, you're going to tell yourself, "Self, this is not the time to worry about that. Self, you're allowed specific times to worry about things *and to work on finding solutions*. But this is not a worry time, so forget it." And just let it go—that is, until the next appropriate time to worry.

This idea sounds simple, yet it can have a major effect on your quality of life. Remind yourself that you need and deserve to sleep well. Remind yourself that worry without action is a waste of energy.

If you still find yourself worrying at bedtime, visualize breathing in through the top of your head and then breathing out the worry and tension through your mouth. And as you lie down, do the bellows breath that's covered in Chapter 11, "Work in Balance." And when you've finished the breathing exercises, relax.

Here's a simple form of meditation you can also use:

Repeat any word or phrase that is comforting to you, such as "Love" or "Peace." Certainly a mantra or religious phrase that is part of your spiritual tradition is appropriate. Pay attention to your breath. When your thoughts wander, bring them gently back to your breath. There are many books available to help you learn meditation. (See Resources.)

Resolve that your time before bed will be a time of peace.

"Now, blessings light on him that first invented this same sleep! It covers a man all over, thoughts and all, like a cloak; it is meat for the hungry, drink for the thirsty, heat for the cold, and cold for the hot. It is the current coin that purchases all the pleasures of the world cheap, and the balance that sets the king and the shepherd, the fool and the wise man, even."

Don Quixote

"Not only does a good night's sleep improve how you feel, it also helps to keep you looking good. It's the all-time, low-cost beauty treatment."

Chapter Eighteen

SLEEP, BLISSFUL SLEEP

The luxury of being able to consistently get a good night's sleep is a hedonist's dream, something pleasurable that descends upon you, without cost or effort. Sleep is what Shakespeare referred to as "great nature's second course, chief nourisher in life's feast."

You just can't beat the cost-benefit ratio of a good night's sleep. Not only does it improve how you feel (because we all know we feel better afterwards), it also helps to keep you looking good. It's the all-time, low-cost beauty treatment!

The challenges of life and the resulting stress can affect your ability to sleep. And not being able to sleep will definitely affect your ability to overcome stress. A vicious cycle develops that leaves you not only tired and irritable, but also with a sense of being dysfunctional. You want to sleep, but you can't.

Or perhaps you often don't have enough hours left for much sleep. You may feel torn between your job and trying to be a good parent. Since you're conscientious about both work and parenting, your only solution so far has been to try to deprive yourself of sleep time.

Excuse the pun, but there are no blanket answers to resolve sleep problems. Your sex, age, job, family, state of health (both mental and physical) and daily stressors will all have a bearing on how you should seek improved sleep. As I mentioned in the last chapter, it's not possible here to present all the ways to improve your sleep. Still, there are generalities that can be made. Some were discussed in the last chapter and you'll find many more in this chapter. You will also learn when the best course of action is to talk to your physician.

A CLOSER LOOK AT SLEEP DEPRIVATION

A lack of sleep can be very harmful. Experiments have shown it to be fatal to mice. We know that it can also be fatal to humans from records of when accidents occur. The industrial accidents at Bhopal, Chernobyl and Three Mile Island all happened after midnight when humans don't function very well. This is also when you are more likely to have a car accident. Interestingly, researchers in Australia found that after 17 hours without sleep, subjects demonstrated the same wakefulness equivalent as that of having a blood alcohol level of 0.05 percent, a level where driving impairments have been documented.

Think of it this way. Your family will not be well served if you fall asleep behind the wheel because you're not getting enough rest. And it could happen. Drowsiness is a major cause of car accidents. According to the U.S. National Traffic Safety Administration, drowsiness may be the cause of approximately 100,000 crashes per year!

A lack of sleep has been shown to affect our immune system. Probably most of us have experienced that; when we've gone through a period of high stress and not enough sleep, we've soon found ourselves sick.

Recently, researchers found that healthy young people

who averaged 6.5 hours of sleep per night had higher insulin resistance than those who averaged 7.5 or 8 hours of sleep. Insulin resistance is a condition that often leads to diabetes. This serious chronic disease is dramatically on the rise in the U.S.

The landmark 1998 study by the National Sleep Foundation found that more than *60 percent* of Americans do not get the recommended eight hours of sleep. And it's getting worse, not better. More than a third of the people surveyed said that the pace of their lives caused them to get less sleep now than they did five years ago. The fact is, we are a nation of sleep-deprived people.

The study also found that women average just 6 hours and 41 minutes of sleep a night. And these sleepless nights were not limited to the months following a child's birth when everyone knows both parents suffer sleep loss. Fifty-six percent, or more than half of the women surveyed, failed to get a good night's sleep due to conditions unique to women, including hormonal fluctuations related to puberty, pregnancy, PMS and perimenopause. And 50 percent more women than men reported that their lack of sleep interfered with their daytime activities.

Further, the study determined that 32 percent of women use medications to help them sleep, compared to just 21 percent of men. Twenty-five percent more women than men reported that they deal with insomnia a few nights a week. Statistically, these are huge numbers.

ARE YOU SLEEP DEPRIVED?

Here are a few of the signs of sleep deprivation:

- Drowsiness after lunch or while driving.
- Falling asleep while you're watching TV or in the bathtub.
- Going to sleep immediately when you go to bed. (It's natural to take approximately 15 minutes to fall asleep.)
- Difficulty concentrating during the day that results in resorting to stimulants such as coffee, sodas, candy bars and cakes/cookies for a boost of energy (very common).
- Finding yourself making frequent mistakes.

POSSIBLE SOLUTIONS
FOR THE OVERWHELMED

If your problem is just not being able to sleep enough because of the demands of your job and family life, that's fortunate in a way. This can be easier to resolve than the problem of someone who is lying awake, night after night, unable to sleep, for the other reasons that will be discussed later in this chapter.

Here are areas to consider if your current responsibilities are leaving you sleep deprived.

If you're staying up late at night to find some peace and quiet, you could try to find it during daylight hours instead. Two ways to do this are by leaving the house to go for a walk, or by taking time on your way home to go to a yoga class. Another possibility is arranging for everyone to be gone simultaneously from the house. Maybe you can swap "peace and quiet weekends" with some of your friends. My brother Bill and his wife found that one of the nicest aspects of Bill's 50th birthday party was that the kids were at their friends' houses the next morning. They actually had a quiet Sunday morning to relax and read the newspaper together as a couple alone.

Are family members helping with housework? You shouldn't be staying up later, or getting up earlier, to do things other family members can pitch in on. Some hints on how to do this: (1) Be very specific about the tasks, (2) Don't nag, (3) Provide lavish praise for the job, even if it's not up to your own standards and (4) Show your appreciation to your mate by being more relaxed and romantic.

And speaking of being relaxed, consider relaxing some of your standards on housework. Your health is more important. Look at it this way. If you become chronically ill, the house could really become a mess. And when your kids are grown, how do you want them to remember you from their childhood—that you were obsessed with housework and a really irritable person to be around, or that you were a relaxed and joyful person?

Finding the happy medium in all of this is not easy, but there's no point in ruining your health for the sake of a clean house. It misses the point. Streamlining routines and making everyone pitch in on weekends is important. Can you hire someone to come in? Can you get rid of a lot of clutter, or assign corners of various rooms, or cabinets, for each person's priceless possessions (that stuff you think of as junk)? Also analyze what you're spending too much time doing and focus on ways to reduce that chunk of time. (See Resources for a book on speed-cleaning.)

Where can you cut corners in the morning routines? If a streamedlined wardrobe, easy hairdos and make-ahead lunch-packing can give you an extra half hour of sleep a night, isn't that worth it?

How much time do you spend commuting? Is there a way for you to work from home a couple of days a week? I know this is a tough question, especially if the boss answers "no." Can you either move closer to your work or can you consider switching jobs? As I said earlier, this book is more about helping you find extra energy to take on tough questions in your life than about actually telling you how to make these decisions. In the meantime, try some of the easier ideas for improving sleep, give yourself some slack, and talk to the people you feel most comfortable with. Hopefully your confidants include your mate, family members or a close friend, but a counselor can also help you come up with creative solutions.

THE SCIENCE OF SLEEP

Before I give you the experts' suggestions for good sleep hygiene, let's review some basic background information. Our bodies have complex metabolic processes that run while we're asleep. For instance, most of the repair work that keeps us functional is done at night. When we deprive ourselves of that time, or make it difficult for the body to do this work, we notice it as fatigue.

Another way to think of this result is in terms of the toxicity of your body. Your liver works to process toxins while you're asleep, and fatigue is a primary symptom of toxicity. So if you're tired all the time, part of it may be that you're impeding this nightly process.

Another important function that happens while we sleep

is the rebuilding of glucose levels that the brain uses for thinking during the day. It's difficult for us to think clearly when we're tired because we have used up the glucose without giving it enough time to replenish.

Sleep is essential to the structural development of our brains when we're babies. It is the time when the brain programs for instinctual behavior are maintained—those things we do without consciously thinking. Sleep is also crucial to the processing and storage of information acquired while we're awake. Our cognitive ability is affected in more than one way if we don't get enough sleep. Albert Einstein used to sleep 11 hours a night. Though the rest of us don't have what he had to start with, any creative endeavor in which you engage, either at work or leisure, will be enhanced by sufficient rest.

Sleep is still a mysterious function. One of the most fascinating areas of brain and sleep research has to do with the role of our dreams and how they affect our individuality. It has been suggested that because we dream, repressive regimes and totalitarianism can never ultimately succeed. This is a powerful thought and should serve to remind you why protecting the space and time where you dream is important to all of us who believe in freedom and individuality. Dreaming is part of what makes you who you are. If anyone questions you about why you insist on a full eight hours' sleep, tell them it's your patriotic duty—you're protecting freedom and individuality. Conversely, sleep deprivation is often used as part of brainwashing strategies.

Among the well-established facts about sleep is that it's normal to have periods of deep sleep, especially early in the night. This is followed by several periods of REM (rapid eye movement) sleep, when dreaming takes place. The REM sleep is interrupted by very brief awakenings. A person with healthy sleep patterns will not be aware of these awakenings, which last only a second or two, and will go back to sleep immediately.

We know our sleep cycles are governed by circadian rhythms. The word "circadian" means "approximately a day." Sleep studies have shown that our natural sleeping/waking cycle is approximately 25 hours long. The studies found that people in a sleep lab, without prompts from daylight, alarm clocks, meals and the morning news, tend to stay up an hour later and sleep an hour later each "day." Over the period of a month, the subjects in these sleep experiments actually lost more than an entire day. For those of us who don't live in sleep labs, this tendency to overrun the daily schedule is reprogrammed every day by sunlight, clocks and work schedules.

GOOD SLEEP HYGIENE TIPS

Out of sleep research comes tips for establishing what is known as "good sleep hygiene." This phrase means establishing and following habits conducive to sleep. While that may sound tedious initially, it can soon become something you're motivated to do without prompting, sort of like brushing your teeth.

Before I describe these ideas, let's pose the question of why you would want to do this instead of taking a pill. Well, a recent study proved that changing your behavior is more effective, as well as safer and non-addictive. A 1999 study on insomnia from Laval University in Quebec found that after two years, many of those who changed their behavior no longer qualified as insomniacs, while those who continued taking medications were still having trouble sleeping.

Now let's look at the tips...

Tip 1. The experts agree that you should get up at the same time every morning, even on weekends. Otherwise, if you stay up very late on Friday and/or Saturday and sleep late on Saturday and/or Sunday, by Monday your brain is confused.

Tip 2. It's very important to get out into sunlight in order to reset your circadian clock to the 24-hour cycle. Bright sunlight going directly to the brain through your eyes in the morning has the effect of overriding the natural human tendency toward a 25-hour day cycle. This argues strongly in favor of the morning walk that you read about in Chapter 7 on walking. If that sounds like torture to you, then compromise by opening blinds as soon as you're vertical. Or if you have a private porch and the weather permits, try having coffee outside in the morning.

Tip 3. Start lowering the amount of artificial light you're exposed to in the evening. Switching from overhead lights to dim table lamps and candles tells your brain that it's nighttime and it will soon be time to sleep.

Tip 4. If you wake up in the middle of the night, try not to turn on any lights. If you're sleepless for more than a half hour and get up, do something very quietly in dim light. If you read, use the least light possible, such as a book light. Turning on bright lights is not going to help you get back to sleep quickly. Nor is turning on the TV or radio, which (depending on the programming) may actually overstimulate you instead of being a calming influence. Reading, stretching or knitting are recommended.

Anyone who has ever knitted will tell you that once you get the hang of it, this is a neat, quiet and very tranquilizing activity. It is being recommended by numerous movie celebrities for its calming effects. (They knit in their trailers between scenes.) I've known that personally for a long time. I credit knitting with helping me get through college successfully. I would knit in all my classes. It kept me from becoming restless.

To my male readers: I recall that Rosey Grier, the famous Los Angeles Rams football player and NFL Hall of Famer, used to do needlework to calm himself. If Grier could do this, so can you. Similarly Jacques Plante, the famous goalie for the Montreal Canadiens hockey team and creator of the mask now worn by all hockey goalies, used needlework to relax. Then again, if you prefer, there's always a book. The important thing is to do what is calming and enjoyable for you. This will help you go back to sleep.

Tip 5. Exercise, but not right before bed. Exercise is critically important, but working out aerobically (such as walking or running) just before bedtime can contribute to difficulty falling asleep. Late afternoon and early evening are excellent times for intense physical activity, but later in the evening, it may cause problems. A few yoga stretches are okay.

Tip 6. Turn the clock away from you so you can't read it from your bed. Experts agree on this. That way, you won't become as frustrated by how long it takes you to fall asleep or return to sleep.

Tip 7. Calm down and relax before you go to bed. The suggestions I've made in the preceding chapters are all part of good sleep hygiene. They have to do with "self-soothing," and letting your brain and your body know that it's time to wind down. Did you ever wonder why those rock stars used to tear up their hotel rooms? Well, it was hard for them to wind down after a performance, especially the drummers. Not that I think the likes of John Bonham or Keith Moon would have taken the suggestion to try an aromatherapy bath. God rest their souls. Instead they just drank themselves to death while their managers paid the hotel repair bills. What a loss! Even if only a few of you truly identify with Bonham and Moon (and you know who you are), it serves to remind you that you need to give yourself some time and healthy ways to unwind. Don't just fall into bed and expect your body to be instantly relaxed. It doesn't work that way.

There are additional steps you can take to help yourself get a better night's sleep.

A *hot bath* will relax your muscles, ease stress symptoms, and also raise your body temperature. Then, when you go to bed, your body temperature will fall again, which is an inducement to sleep. Conversely, when your body temperature rises, it can wake you up, as women with hot flashes often report.

For the same reason, a *cool room* is more likely to help you fall asleep than a warm one. The body's temperature is naturally slightly lower during sleep. If you become overly warm, you may wake up. It may be one of the reasons many people like to sleep with a window open. You do want your feet to be warm, however. If you have cold feet, socks are probably a good idea. You might try a hot water bottle for your feet. Another way to use a hot water bottle is to place it right over your liver (on your right side, just below the rib cage). Your liver works at a slightly higher temperature than the rest of your body. A hot water bottle saves the liver the energy it would expend to achieve that slightly higher temperature and allows it to be that much more effective.

Besides, this is very comforting.

The temperature of the room, weight of sleeping apparel and the number of blankets, or lack of them, is very individual. It is, however, an easy aspect to experiment with, unless your mate has dramatically different preferences.

If you're anxious, *reading books of a calming nature* before you go to bed can be very helpful. It doesn't matter what your favorite books might be, the point is to read the books and allow yourself to be relaxed by them.

If you have problems sleeping, your choices of food and beverage may be a factor. I won't tell you that you can't eat or drink your favorites, but it may help to learn *when* would be a better time to consume them.

Eating a heavy meal late at night is not healthy. I used to hear this said, but I never understood why until I learned about detox. Now I know. Basically, your liver has things it needs to be doing in the middle of the night other than digesting the food it thinks you should have eaten hours earlier. It can't do everything at once. If you don't allow the liver to do its detox work, you're creating a time bomb for your health. For this reason, a big bowl of ice cream right before bed is not a good choice, either of food or of timing. You'd be better off with a baked potato with a little olive oil or low fat yogurt as a topping. Regardless of the time you eat them, high-fat foods add an extra load onto the liver, which supplies the bile that is needed to break fats down to fatty acids. That wisecrack remark, "Why bother to eat it? Why not apply it directly to the waistline?" is especially true about eating high-fat foods late at night.

Many people find that indigestion wakes them in the middle of the night. My advice is to reconsider the information about food strategies in Chapter 9 because those

PROGRESSIVE RELAXATION

A stress-reduction technique called progressive relaxation can be helpful in falling asleep or returning to sleep. It's simple to do in bed.

- Lie on your back, arms at your sides.
- Raise your right leg slightly above the bed and tense it as hard as you can for four seconds. Hold your breath while you tense your leg. Then let it drop and let go of the breath. Repeat with your left leg.
- Next tense your buttocks as hard as you can for four seconds, while holding your breath. Then relax.
- Next, take a big breath and tense your chest. Hold it. Then relax.
- Raise your arms slightly above the bed. Tense them really hard, while holding your breath. Then relax.
- Turn your head gently from side to side a couple of times, breathing in and out.
- Then, scrunch up your face like a prune. Hold it. Then relax.
- Let your chin drop, stick out your tongue and try to make your face as long as possible.
- Now observe how relaxed you feel.

Go back to your feet mentally. Say to yourself, "My feet are going to be completely relaxed." Repeat it. Then say to yourself, "My feet are now completely relaxed," and mentally scan your feet, letting go of any tension. In succession, do the same with your lower legs, upper legs, buttocks, shoulders, arms, neck, face and brain.

Then scan your entire body for any tightness and focus your breath on that spot and tell that spot to relax. Tell yourself to let go of all the tension, anywhere in your body. If you're still awake at this point, slowly and gently shift to your favorite sleeping position and focus on your breathing.

ideas can help prevent indigestion as well as promote higher energy levels and loss of weight. The simple concept of fruit first thing in the morning followed by protein-dense foods midday and carbohydrates mostly at night is a powerful one.

If you have problems sleeping, *stop drinking coffee after lunch*. The issue of caffeine in coffee is rather well-known, but there are also other sources of caffeine that are hidden. Many medications contain caffeine, both the prescription type and over-the-counter product. Ask your pharmacist for advice. Also hot chocolate, tea and many soft drinks contain caffeine. Read the labels.

To help yourself relax, there are *herb teas* you can sip before bed. If you find this causes you to have to wake to urinate during the night, you might want to drink the tea an hour or two before bedtime.

One tea to consider is *chamomile*, an excellent after-dinner choice because it is also a digestive aid. Chamomile is very safe and available in the tea section of just about any supermarket. Warning: If you are allergy-prone, it might cause a reaction. One way you'll know is if you sneeze when you open the package.

Another tea is *valerian root* (*Valeriana officinalis*), which is considered a mild sedative. You'll need to continue drinking the valerian tea for a couple of weeks before you can be sure whether it's working. Many people add lemon juice or orange peel if they don't find the taste appealing. Like many herbal remedies, valerian has been used therapeutically for thousands of years. Also, as with other herbs, it can be taken in different forms, either as a tea, in capsules or in a tincture. (The capsules avoid the issue of taste, and the tincture can be diluted in a small glass of water and swallowed in a gulp.) The personnel at the health food store can direct you to all three products, which may not be in the same spot in the store. Follow the package instructions on usage. Valerian does not create any "hangover" or grogginess the next day, but still requires respect. It can interact with medications such as benzodiazepines (including Xanax). Like other sedatives, when taken in large doses, valerian can be fatal.

Other sleep-inducing herbal preparations can be found at the health food store. They may include ingredients such as lemon balm (*Melissa officinalis*) and catnip (*Nepeta cataria*), both gentle enough to be found in children's formulas. Skullcap (*Scutellaria laterifolia*) is classified as a sedative, and it's often used to calm nervous tension. Passionflower (*Passiflora incarnata*) is yet another herb with sedative as well as hypnotic effects. Hops (*Humulus lupulus*), well known as an ingredient in beer, has similar effects, though it is contraindicated for those also suffering from depression. A trained herbalist could recommend a customized blend, or you could experiment cautiously with the commercial blends you find at the health food store.

If you're on medication, you should always check with your physician before using any herb for therapeutic purposes. Doctors are becoming more knowledgeable about herbs, though some of them are still naysayers. Finding a holistically oriented physician is the best of both worlds. More of these special health care professionals are becoming available, but unfortunately there are still not enough to go around.

Make sure you're taking a *calcium citrate and magnesium supplement.* This combination is not only important to help prevent osteoporosis; it also enhances one's ability to fall asleep.

While we're talking about supplements, *melatonin* has become very popular in the past few years. Melatonin is a hormone produced naturally by the body between the hours of midnight and 3 a.m. There has been a great deal written about melatonin recently. It has been called a "cure for jet lag," a claim that seems to be substantiated by follow-up research.

Other claims have been made that melatonin slows aging and restores vitality. Melatonin has also been touted as a sleep aid. Research is still being conducted, and it's too early to tell if all the claims will be validated. In my own experience, melatonin seemed to contribute to vivid dreams, which was interesting, like going to see a movie, but it also left me a bit groggy the next morning. It could be worth a try if you take melatonin carefully. Remember that it is a hormone and might cause undesirable side effects if used in very high quantities. Start with a low dose, 0.3 to 0.5 milligrams, which might mean that you have to break apart a capsule. Check with your doctor if you have a chronic disease, especially an autoimmune condition.

It's a common misconception that an *alcoholic drink* will help you sleep. Although it may help you fall asleep, it may also wake you up. Alcohol is a form of sugar; as the alcohol is metabolized, it will increase the level of glucose in your bloodstream, possibly causing you to wake up. Obviously, *eating sweets* before you go to bed will also cause your blood sugar to spike.

Drinking alcohol late at night also interferes with the liver's functioning, so a nightcap is not a good way to help you sleep. Also, alcohol tends to aggravate snoring.

A SOLUTION FOR SNORING

A simple herbal tea is proving quite effective against snoring. Make a cup of cinnamon tea, add two teaspoons of grated ginger, plus honey and milk to taste, and drink the tea each night before bed. This is cheaper than surgery and those nose strips too. Ginger is also a wonderful liver cleanser, so it can help you or your mate in more than one way.

Smoking late at night is also not advised as a way to help you fall asleep. One reason is that nicotine stimulates adrenaline production. I know this could be a difficult choice. If you want to put off tackling that addiction, I understand. Try some of the other suggestions mentioned here. If nothing else works, try Hall's® Sugar Free Mentholyptus Cough Drops for a couple of nights instead of a cigarette before you go to bed, or if you wake up. The menthol in Hall's Cough Drops is so strong that you can take a "drag" on it the same way you do on a cigarette. It's worth a try to see if it will help you to sleep better.

SLEEPING GEAR & MORE

If you're sensitive to noise, *earplugs* can help you to sleep more comfortably. They can both block sounds present as you're falling asleep as well as noise generated during the night (such as from someone returning home after you've gone to bed).

Have you been sleeping on a really old and sagging *mattress*? Then purchasing a new one is probably a good idea. A good mattress should last about 10 years. If the price seems high, try this. Amortize the amount out over that period of time and think how important a good night's rest is on a daily basis. You'll see that this is not an expensive investment, no matter how much you spend.

Buying a mattress is not particularly easy. Mattresses are a hard thing to ask advice about, because this is a very individual choice. However, you can ask your friends if they like theirs and what brand and model they are. Then ask if you can just test it a bit. (This may trigger a laugh or at least a smile or two.) If you sleep on a hotel mattress that you find particularly comfortable, make a note of the name of the manufacturer. If this is not on the mattress label, the hotel staff may be able to determine the name. Two websites are listed in Resources that may be helpful in making a decision. Unfortunately, a lot of shopping may be involved in finding the right mattress for you. Make up your mind not to rush into a decision. You don't want to spend a lot on a mattress that doesn't improve your sleep.

HEALTH PROBLEMS & SLEEP

We need good sleep as much when we age as when we are young. However, we naturally tend to sleep less as we age. And we tend to become sleepy earlier, and then wake up earlier—like four o'clock in the morning! Other natural biological changes contribute to making it more difficult to sleep well. These include hot sweats during menopause, an overactive bladder or prostate problems (which can cause a man to have to get up in the middle of the night to urinate). Pain from arthritis or fibromyalgia often interrupts sleep.

If your sleep difficulties don't begin to noticeably improve after you've implemented several of the behavioral suggestions listed earlier in this chapter, it's important to talk to your doctor. Perhaps your inclination is just to try over-the-counter (OTC) sleep medications and see if they can help. The problem is that the ingredients that cause drowsiness in OTC preparations are antihistamines formulated primarily to reduce nasal congestion. Drowsiness is one of their side effects. If you're having sleep problems, your physician can provide a more appropriate medication.

There are other, more severe health problems that affect the quality of sleep, and your sleeplessness could be a symptom of one of them. These include:

- Alzheimer's disease
- Anemia
- Angina
- Anxiety
- Asthma
- Chronic obstructive pulmonary disease
- Coronary artery disease
- Depression
- Hypertension
- Irregular heartbeat
- Obstructive sleep apnea
- Parkinson's disease
- Underactive or overactive thyroid

The most common of these among women is depression, which can rob not only you but also your family, of much of the joy of living. Depression can be a life-threatening condition. The good news is that treatment for depression has progressed very rapidly. Most healthcare practitioners recognize it as a biochemical imbalance, and they also see how important it is to treat depression efficiently, before it leads to other physical health problems. New medications as well as new approaches to talk therapy are very effective for most people. Help is available. Don't try to bootstrap yourself out of a depression if it has lasted more than three or four months. Make an appointment, and don't make your healthcare provider guess what your problem is. If your provider can't help you, ask for a referral to a mental healthcare specialist. If your provider won't refer you, call your insurance company and find out what your coverage is for mental health treatment. It varies widely depending on state law. Then ask for a referral. If you have no insurance, call information and ask for a number for your local County Department of Mental Healthcare (or something similar). They can help.

Meanwhile, don't let up on your healthy hedonist activities. It can take a while before the biochemical improvements these activities generate will be noticeable, but give them a chance. They're all based on clinically proven, preventive health measures. I've compiled the ideas in this book to make sure you're not only more healthy, but having a better time as well. And if you didn't believe that was important, I don't think you would have made it this far in the book!

Part Three

Weekend Pleasures

*"Give me books, fruit, French wine and fine weather
and a little music out of doors,
played by someone I do not know."*

John Keats

"If you find you have too much to do, there are ways to stretch the weekend by combining a few activities."

Chapter Nineteen

GOOD, BETTER, BEST WEEKENDS

Weekends are those days when you try to cram in all the rest, relaxation, exercise, fun, adventure and familial togetherness that you can't become involved in during the week. It's also a time you have to do things to get ready for the next work-week. And don't forget those "few" home maintenance or remodeling details on your list. These usually aren't tackled on a weekday.

A quick assessment indicates that unless you live alone in a sparse apartment or condo, have no nearby relatives, and do very little or none of your own cooking, you tend to have an overload of expectations for those two precious days at the end of the week. I now vaguely remember those years when the only thing I *had* to do on Sunday was read the newspaper. Now, on some weekends, I feel lucky if I get through the "A" section.

Fortunately, without becoming overstressed about it, I usually find there are ways to stretch the weekend. My strategy is to combine a few activities.

MARKETING IN MOTION

The first strategy is to combine exercise and shopping in ways that are more fun than just going to a grocery and a gym. I have to give credit to my dogs for inspiring this approach. But you can also take your kids. It works about the same.

Start by finding the location of your local *farmers' markets*. These have become very popular in the past few years because they provide opportunities to buy the freshest produce, often for less than you pay at conventional supermarkets. Even if it turns out to be a bit more expensive, it's money well spent. It goes directly to the farmer, and you're buying better produce.

Generally farmers' markets are set up in large parking lots, or in an area where a couple of streets are blocked off for a few hours. It's an outdoor environment, with a mood and pace so different from a grocery store that you can't help feeling like you've gone to a fair. You can enhance the feeling by wearing an interesting wide-brimmed hat, which not only protects your skin, but makes you part of the scenery as well. By buying fresh flowers at the market, you can bring that festive mood back home with you.

Besides produce and flowers, there are usually vendors selling craft items, homemade breads, honey, nuts and an interesting mix of other products. There are often musicians busking for donations from the crowd. Some food or beverage vendors are usually on hand, cooking up ethnic delights or offering coffee drinks. People bring their kids and stroll around. Plan to take a little extra time so you can enjoy food or a beverage while you're there.

It's a great place to meet a friend, so you can then do three things at once—shop, exercise and socialize. And there's no charge for admission!

You usually have to park a little farther away than you would from a grocery store, so this is where some of the exercise comes in. It might be a good idea to bring a little cart, and definitely a lot of cloth or mesh shopping bags. You'll know after your first time or two how much you tend to buy. I used to purchase 25-pound sacks of organic oranges and not much else because that was all I could carry. I'd just throw a bag over my shoulder as though I were a longshoreman and walk the two blocks back to the office, wearing a skirt and stockings. This was before I switched to pantsuits.

Most markets don't allow you to bring your dogs into the actual area of the market for health reasons. But I've been known to plan my trip to coincide with a trip to a dog park, where both the dogs and I are able to do a fair amount of walking and running around. The dogs are pretty quiet after that and I can leave them in the car, in the shade, with the windows partially down so it doesn't become too warm for them. On a "dog day," I never dillydally over coffee. It's more like a commando raid at the market. Get in, get out and get home.

How do you find a farmers' market? They are generally sponsored by a city, so you could begin with the public information officer at City Hall. An activities office is another place to ask, as well as the Convention and Visitors Bureau or tourist information office. Don't give up without calling the reference desk at the public library. Librarians are intelligent and very helpful people, as well as fantastic at figuring out where information is stored. A little Internet searching might be the easiest way. Do an advanced search on "farmers' market" and the name of your town. If nothing pops up, try the names of adjacent towns.

While you're at it, search on *Community-supported Agriculture* and the name of your state. This can be another fun and adventurous way to shop.

Community-supported agriculture (CSA) is an important trend for encouraging small organic farms. It works like this. A group of families pledge to underwrite a farmer's cost. They pay at least a portion of this money in advance, and the farmer knows that he has a market for the food he grows. The families, in turn, receive very high-quality organic produce, which they receive on a weekly basis during the summer and early autumn months. Sometimes there is such an abundance that the question of exactly how to preserve the produce until it can be eaten comes into play. But there is also the delight of seeing how much fresh produce you can actually eat. Huge salads, great mounds of fresh steamed spinach and wondrous stir fries are some of the results.

But the families also receive something else that's very important. Through their farmer, they have a link to the land, to the work and to the people who bring food to their table. Most of us have become divorced from the actual processes of growing food. We walk into a grocery store and it's all laid out there for us, with no hint as to what it takes to provide what is still the most important product of human endeavor. Food. We don't get anything done without it.

Community-supported agriculture is a symbiotic system that is helping to protect farm land. We not only have a tremendous need to preserve this land for the pure, plain necessity of having a place where we CAN grow food, but also because farm land fosters the wildlife that nibbles at the edges.

CSA plans vary from place to place. Some provide organic produce while others don't. You might make your payments weekly or monthly. Another variable is whether you go to the farm to pick up your produce or have it delivered. (In some plans, delivery is extra.) Going to the farm makes this even more of a community event, where you can get to know the farm staff and other CSA participants. Some farms have surplus tables where members leave items they don't want. At this table, you may find yourself swapping items with a new friend. Driving out into the country, you're also likely to find a perfect spot for a stroll.

You could create an equivalent by finding a farm fresh produce stand that you can frequent regularly. Get to know the people. Ask questions. Show some interest. And while you're away from home, look for new areas for your walks. Then get moving and enjoy the change in scenery from your neighborhood jaunts.

In addition, *growing food in your own backyard* is a great way to get your food and exercise simultaneously. But I won't kid you. It's a lot of work. I think you already know if you have an interest in gardening or not. If you do, but don't have a yard or it isn't large enough, look around for a community garden. Or call the Cooperative Extension office for your county (every county has one) and ask if they have a number for the Master Gardeners program. The Master Gardeners program trains volunteer gardeners to provide advice and assistance to other people who are learning to garden. Their office can direct you to a nearby community garden, help you find out if plots are available and also provide advice on every aspect of growing your own produce. Though gardening is lots of work, it is marvelously therapeutic. It is calming and gives you perspective. The plants respond to your love and attention.

EXERCISING & SOCIALIZING

I want to cautiously throw out the word "hike" here. But I'm doing it cautiously because I don't want you to get the idea that I'm talking about backpacking in the mountains. I'm talking more about taking advantage of a regional park, a river bank or some other area that's close by where you can walk and enjoy the natural environment.

The advantage of walking-based forms of exercise is that you can talk while you're in motion. Walking with a friend or with family then becomes an enjoyable social activity.

You can combine walking with a picnic and this can become a memorable occasion. Picnics were a favorite activity of my family when I was young and I've never lost my appreciation for them. In fact, it has increased. When you put a nice bottle of wine in the picnic basket, some good bread and cheese, some fresh fruit and a couple of squares of chocolate, it's a gourmet delight.

When I went to Italy a few years ago with my mother and sister, we refined our picnics. That wasn't hard, being in Italy. Since then, the three of us have each acquired our own picnic backpacks that have all the supplies for a stylish picnic—tablecloth, napkins, plastic wine glasses, plates, utensils and, of course, the corkscrew. It's nice to have it all together because you can grab it and go, with just one stop at the deli.

Our new personal favorites for the picnic basket are little jars of roasted eggplant in olive oil. Running a close second is black olive paste. Either of those on crackers is delicious all by itself, but we invented a great *hors d'oeuvre*—a cracker with first a little black olive paste, then a slice of mozzarella cheese and finally a slice of tomato.

A lot of my picnicking in Southern California takes place

at the Hollywood Bowl. With 17,000 seats, the Bowl attracts world-class entertainment. The great news is that the seats in the back sell for about five dollars. There's absolutely nothing wrong with the sound in those seats, you just can't see what's happening on onstage very well unless you bring binoculars. But you can get a mild aerobic workout getting to your seat.

Summer events with festival seating have become very popular. If you're not in the habit of taking advantage of them, consider attending one of these events. They offer an opportunity to combine a bit of exercise with a great deal of pleasure.

SHARE YOUR IDEAS

I'm sure there are dozens of ways that I haven't personally experienced to combine great fun with mild exercise and sociability, so I look forward to receiving any suggestions you have. To send your ideas, visit our website, *www.thehealthyhedonist.com*, or email them to me—janet@thehealthyhedonist.com.

"If you don't have the energy to wash and chop veggies, ask yourself, do I have the energy to just wash and fit them in the juicer? Because that's all it takes, really. "

Chapter Twenty

JUICING & SATURDAY SALADS

THE JOY OF JUICING

Have you noticed how much better fresh-squeezed orange juice *tastes* compared to the frozen variety? The juice is also a lot better for you when it's fresh.

Juicing extracts the most nutritious elements of fresh fruits and vegetables. A person who drinks raw juice absorbs an amazing 99 percent of the vitamins, minerals, trace minerals, antioxidants and phytonutrients contained in those fresh fruits and vegetables. This happens, because juice—by virtue of being a liquid—can be quickly and easily absorbed by the body. This eliminates, or circumvents, all sorts of problems that some people have digesting raw fruits and vegetables.

When you drink fresh juice on an empty stomach—such as first thing in the morning, or mid-morning or mid-afternoon—the nutrients will be in your bloodstream within 10 minutes. This will provide a lift that's genuinely nutritious.

I find that juicing appeals to people who aren't wild about salads. My husband is one of them. Patrick eats salads, but he's not crazy about them. But he loves juices. And Patrick isn't the only one who appreciates the results. My dogs like the pulp. Okay, they're unusual. Bo and Boogie also like "carrot-bones" and cabbage leaves.

Here's a little more good news about juicing. You don't have to be terribly proficient with a knife and chopping board to easily and competently make juice. And it requires little energy. In the evening, if you don't have the energy to wash and finely chop a lot of veggies for a stir fry or salad, ask yourself, do I have the energy to just wash and slice them enough to fit in the juicer? Because that's all it takes, really. You don't need many ingredients for a juice blend— two or three is plenty. (If you add too many, you can't discern the taste of the individual ingredients.) A blend of two or three ingredients makes an excellent cocktail before dinner, one the whole family can indulge in, any night of the week.

Fresh juicing educates your palate to the flavors and delicacy of "live" foods. Keep in mind that fresh juice deteriorates very rapidly, just the way a fresh salad does.

You've been taught to think that bottled and frozen juices are healthy, but they really aren't, compared to fresh juice. Bottled juices are pasteurized to kill microbes that naturally grow in fresh food exposed to air, or that remain on the skin of produce from the growing, picking, packing and shipping processes. For public safety, we agree that's a good thing. Food poisoning can be deadly. But pasteurization also kills the enzymes and most of the vitamins, which are some of the most healthful aspects of the juice.

The care that goes into juicing at home doesn't happen in a commercial canning operation. For example, you carefully wash fruit before juicing, cut out the bad spots, immediately juice the fruit and then enjoy the drink. This means that air-borne microbes do not have a chance to multiply.

The process of commercial bottling also causes oxidation. Fresh apple juice is white, like the inside of an apple. Bottled apple juice is brown, due to oxidation. There are also high quantities of mold in bottled juices, because juice manufacturers don't carefully pick out moldy fruit the way you would at home. You may not be able to taste it, but that mold adds an extra load that your immune system must carry. If your immune system is in any way compromised—and to a certain extent, all of ours are compromised by the chemicals in the environment—it's best to avoid foods that tax your body unnecessarily. True, bottled juice is more healthy than soda pop (because it doesn't have the chemical additives that sodas do), but bottled juice is *less* healthy than plain filtered water. Why? Well, the bottled juice is high in natural sugar, without giving you all of the enzymes and vitamins of fresh juice. A good compromise is flavored waters.

If you've never been into juicing, and don't have a juicer, you can begin this fresh fruits and vegetables adventure by checking out a juice bar or two. I suggest you find one near your home or work. You'll discover a wide array of choices. If you don't have an immediate preference, ask the counter help what's popular, which of the fruits are freshest and what juices are their own personal favorites. They have probably tried almost everything in the store.

Make a point to notice the taste of the juice and then pay attention to how you feel after you drink it. The fresh juice should give you an immediate energy pick-me-up and leave you feeling refreshed from the inside out.

For now, stay away from smoothies made with ice cream, sorbet or sherbet. You're in the process of educating your pallet to the taste and effect of real, fresh juice. Ice cream, sorbet and sherbet have a lot of processed sugar added. Later in the chapter, I'll tell you more about making delicious and healthy sherbets, sorbets and fruit "puddings" at home.

A good *juicer* is a smart investment. You'll want to take some time to research their various features and benefits, relative to cost. Meanwhile, you might want to buy a little electric *citrus juicer*, which is quite inexpensive. They cost around $20 to $25. That minor investment will allow you to begin to develop a fresh fruit juice habit by making fresh orange and grapefruit juices. Try different combinations. When tangerines are in season, they make a very special treat. Blood oranges, when you can find them, will add color.

You'll want to have a citrus juicer anyway. It's a good choice for juicing on weekday mornings, because there's much less work in setting up and cleaning it. You can juice and "drink" several oranges in two or three minutes. It would take you much longer to peel and eat them.

Your next minor investment could be a *book on juicing*. I say this because it's inspirational. The number of combinations for juicing are limitless, and just to read the recipes will make your mouth water. I hesitate to start naming combinations because they might be my favorites and not yours. Just think of one fruit you like, then think of another, think of combining them, then add something else for color and zest. You could combine the juice with sparkling mineral water and serve it over ice; this is especially refreshing on a hot afternoon. Watermelon juice over ice is fantastic. Any melon can be juiced very easily and is wonderfully cooling in summer.

Tropical fruits are fabulous additions to basic juices such as apple or orange. For example, fresh orange with pineapple is wonderful. Serve it over ice with lime and it's even tastier and more refreshing. When you can find them, guava and/or passion fruit are wonderful with orange juice.

A small quantity of cranberries will perk up any other fruit and they can be bought inexpensively during the holidays. Tip: you can store cranberries in the freezer for months. You don't need to defrost them—just throw a few in with the rest of the ingredients.

A great thing about juicing is that you can combine fruits and vegetables in juices that you would never think of mixing in a salad. A few surprising but delicious combinations are pineapple, radishes and celery. Or oranges, spinach and parsley. Or red cabbage and pineapple. That last combination might not sound good, but trust me on it. It not only has a nice sweet-tart taste, but the color is phenomenal. It's a beautifully frothy reddish purple.

Cabbage is very healthy and affordable, but otherwise, how much of it would you want to eat? I like cole slaw as well as the next person, but I only want to eat it occasionally. The surprising thing is that cabbage juice makes a great base ingredient in juicing. If the cabbage is fresh, you can barely tell it's cabbage when you juice it. And as soon as you add other ingredients to it, you can't detect any cabbage taste. Plus, as I mentioned, since juice is so digestible, you don't have any of the problems commonly associated with cabbage. In addition, cabbage has important nutritional benefits. For instance, it has a lot of the amino acid, glutathione. While cabbage juice might not be the first one you will want to experiment with, once you're feeling a bit braver, give it a try.

Carrots are a mainstay of juicing. Carrot juice tastes much better than cooked carrots and it's incredibly good for you. It's also quite sweet tasting. My favorite carrot juice combinations are with beet juice and ginger root, which is spicy, or with apple juice. Cucumber mellows it out, making it less sweet. Carrots are also great juiced with pineapple or orange juice.

Tip: I find that juicing is a good way to quickly use fruits that are becoming overly ripe.

A good juicer will cost at least a couple of hundred dollars, and certain types go up to $500. But think of it as an investment in good health. Ask yourself how much health insurance costs, or what some people have to spend every month on medication. Then you can start to put the price into perspective. Many of the juicing books tell you how to use juice therapeutically. I like to think of it as one of the best and ultimately easiest health habits you can possibly develop.

There are three secrets to easy juicing:

1. Purchase a juicer that is easier to clean.
2. Purchase one that is simple to use.
3. Keep the juicer out on the counter, along with the other appliances you use every day.

Another way to become a fresh-juice maker is to look for a used juicer through classified ads, garage sales, on the bulletin board at the health store or perhaps on eBay. I won't say that a good used one is just as good as a new one, but I've had a couple of used ones that did the job. And I certainly couldn't complain about how much I'd spent on them.

I now have a Champion® juicer. It's rather large and virtually indestructible. It features a well-constructed motor and a couple of simple attachments that are easy to clean. It ejects the pulp as the juice is made. This is an important detail. Other juicers have to be cleaned during the juicing process if you're making more than a little juice.

SORBETS, SHERBETS & PUDDINGS

The Champion juicer can also be used to create sorbets, sherbets and puddings. The booklet that comes with the machine uses the term "homogenize" to describe the process. Never mind if you don't understand how it works. The result is what's important and that's sorbets, banana "pudding" desserts and all sorts of concoctions that are tasty and nutritious. When compared to the fat and calories of most desserts, they're a "steal." If you need an extra selling point for investing in a Champion juicer, the fact that it makes great desserts could be it. Ask someone at a health food store to show you the booklet that comes with the juicer. Meanwhile, if you know how to use blenders and other kitchen equipment to achieve the same effects, please let me know at *www.thehealthyhedonist.com.*

THE SATURDAY SALAD

Here's a way to maximize some of your weekend produce preparation time. On Saturday, make a salad big enough for two days. Make sure you tear the lettuce leaves rather than cut them. And make sure you've dried them well in a salad spinner or a clean dish towel. These steps prevent the leaves from turning brown rapidly. If you store the salad in a well-sealed plastic container, this also helps it to stay fresh.

Divide the salad into two different bowls. Just pour dressing on one half on Saturday and leave the second half covered in the refrigerator until the next day. Ingredients that will store well for at least a day are lettuce, sliced radishes, celery, sliced cucumber, chopped green onions and slivers of red cabbage. There are certain ingredients you wouldn't want to use with this approach, including sprouts, tomatoes, strong onions and avocados. These ingredients can be quickly and easily added the next day, along with fun and tasty ingredients such as sunflower seeds and croutons.

This concept came to me when I stayed the weekend at the house of friends. For dinner, my hostess made a wonderful salad with watercress, grapes, candied pecans and shallots. There was plenty of salad left. We saved it for the next day when I had it for breakfast; the flavors were sweet and delicate. I could have eaten it with lunch or dinner, but I thought it made an outstanding breakfast. All those greens helped detox the wine I'd imbibed the night before.

I mention this last concept as a way of suggesting that you abandon food conventionalities and figure out what *works* for you. And hopefully, you'll consider sharing the approaches you develop with the rest of us at *www.thehealthyhedonist.com!*

"With coordination, you can make three or four dishes in a session and have home-cooked meals all week with only one kitchen session. Think of it as a party, not a chore. "

Chapter Twenty-One

COOKING WITH FAMILY & FRIENDS

Close to 46 million women in the U.S. now work full-time outside the home. The ramifications for our society and culture are vast. Sociologists will keep busy for decades figuring them out.

But here is something we already know—among the changes is less time spent cooking. A recent study found that, on average, the U.S. family spends only one-half hour a day preparing meals. It's rather easy to derive from that figure that not too many families are sitting down to freshly cooked meals every evening. No criticism intended. Who wants to have to wait an hour to eat after arriving home brain-dead and dog-tired. And not only that, to also be expected to find energy for cooking. I even know of a woman who went house-hunting for a home *without* a kitchen. That's how much she didn't cook!

As a result of the changes, there has been a corresponding increase in meals eaten "out," whether in a restaurant, at a fast food place, or even on the run. Restaurant meals now make up 60 percent of food budgets. Additionally, the market for frozen entrees, supermarket "deli" foods and other no-cook or easy-to-cook foods has grown enormously.

All this would be fine, but there is a direct correlation

between all those meals eaten out and the soaring rates for obesity and diabetes. Most prepared foods, most food served in restaurants and almost all fast food is high in fat and carbohydrates, as well as loaded with preservatives and other additives.

Meanwhile all the research on maintaining weight and preventing chronic degenerative diseases reaffirms the need to eat right-fat foods and lots of FRESH fruits and vegetables. But unless you eat out at a salad bar every night, how are you going to achieve that?

I can only tell you what works for me. Convenience is one of the reasons I make sure to eat two to three pieces of fruit every morning. It means that before 9 a.m., I'm well on my way to meeting the suggested quota of at least five servings of fresh fruit and vegetables a day.

Making cooking fun is another important element of the strategy I use to turn fresh vegetables into tasty meals. At least once a week, I try to cook a somewhat larger quantity of food that I can then freeze.

PARTY, PARTY

Parties give me energy. I love the whole process of preparing for a dinner party, from the planning to the shopping, cleaning the house, prettying everything up, then the cooking and scurrying to have everything ready at the same time, including myself. I even love cleaning up after a party, because I'm still savoring the event, the leftovers and the last drop of wine. I actually like to carefully wash the special dishes I've brought out for the event, gradually clearing the table until only the flowers and candles remain, all the while listening to music.

I also love to eat party food for a couple of days after.

Having enough left over so that I don't have to cook is a bonus to having the party in the first place. Of course, the idea is to plan foods that are high in vegetables and lower in fat so I won't feel guilty about eating the foods that remain.

You might think from those statements that I do a lot of entertaining. I don't. But when I do, I always look forward to it for weeks and even months.

COOK-A-THONS WITH FAMILY & FRIENDS

Like most people who enjoy cooking, I learned by helping my mother. As a result, I'm oriented to team cooking. I find that when I'm with family, cooking is easy and natural—something that happens almost effortlessly while we all catch up on each other's lives and ideas.

If you have family nearby, it's easy to make family visits an excuse for doing enough cooking so there's something to freeze for dinners during the following week. Or you may have a friend nearby who enjoys cooking. The two of you can consider creating a cooking team. Even a cook-a-thon once a month can be a pleasant occasion that results in *"planned-overs."* These dishes, when reheated and served with a salad, some steamed veggies, or even a glass of fresh squeezed juice, yield a well-balanced meal. Reheating works especially well with soups and stews, which are both excellent ways to incorporate vegetables into your diet. They aren't fresh by the time you eat them, but they started out fresh. That means that the fiber, and most of the vitamin and mineral content, has been captured in the liquids. Plus you know what else went into it and what didn't (no preservatives, no extra salt, just plain good ingredients).

There's also the Tender Loving Care component. A meal made of nutritious ingredients by someone who loves you and savored with loving friends and family definitely meets more than physical needs.

Here's yet another reason for cooking at home that you'll understand. I enjoy eating in restaurants as much as the next person, but have you ever seen those scenes in TV reports and movies about what goes on in restaurant kitchens, especially if you send the food back? And thank goodness for health department regulations. Otherwise, what goes on in restaurant kitchens would be much worse.

Cooking at home is important to your health for a lot of reasons. So figuring out fun ways to make it happen is definitely a good idea.

Back to the cook-a-thon: What if you knew that you could have home-cooked meals all week and that it would only take one kitchen session to make this happen? This would benefit not only your health, but your pocketbook as well. What could you do with the savings?

With a bit of coordination, if there's more than one of you cooking, you can make three or four different dishes in a session. Instead of chopping onions four times, one of you chops onions once, etc. It's an occasion that makes it worthwhile to pull out the food processor and the other kitchen gadgets you may rarely use. The kitchen might get warm, but the assembled family or household members will love it. Think of it as a party, not a chore. You'll be loose and well-fed at the end of dinner, with meals to use for days.

In the warm months, the cook-a-thon is a barbeque. Though the menu is different, the idea is the same. And you're more likely to be able to enlist additional friends or family members in the cooking and grilling activities. Barbeque food that makes good planned-overs includes a wide array of grilled meats and vegetables plus all kinds of cold and marinated salads. Summer soups, served cold, also store well. (Barbequing more often than once a week cannot be considered healthy, so this idea only works on an occasional basis.)

If your kitchen is small, or you just prefer to cook all by yourself, a similar idea is to do dinner parties with a close friend. Both of you can cook alone for the same party, but make enough so that you each have planned-overs of all the entrees. A phone call to compare recipes and menus before hand ensures that you're not each cooking something similar. It's a good way to try new recipes as well as old favorites.

Slightly more involved is to just have a dinner party circle with three or four friends.

Meals are meant to be social occasions. I realize that's becoming the exception rather than the rule, but it shouldn't be impossible.

I know you've seen it in movies—the Italian family eating together around a big table, everyone talking loudly and gesturing, while the cooks (usually the women, but not always) bring in huge plates of food from the kitchen. If this is not something you come by naturally as a result of your own personal or cultural heritage, it's something you can mimic. And if it wouldn't be any fun with your family of origin, create a family of friends who would make this a joyful celebration.

My parents showed us that there is no finer entertainment than dinner with friends, and nothing so comfortable as dinner at home. When my father was home (Dad traveled a lot), he would almost always have a cocktail before dinner. My dad is a very witty, jovial person by nature and he'd often have a joke to tell. His delivery was great, but usually it was his own enjoyment of the joke that was funnier than the content.

Frequently one of his friends would come over. Our two favorites were an architect, a man who we "adopted" as our "godfather," and my father's other close friend, a judge we also enjoyed immensely. The judge and my dad were both crazy about golf and liked to go on golfing vacations with their wives, especially in Portugal and Mexico. The judge was from an old Hispanic family and spoke the most beautiful Spanish I've ever heard. There was a wealth of storytelling and laughter on the evenings when either the architect or the judge came by. They would have a couple of drinks with my father and stay for a full meal before driving safely home.

My father taught us that being rich is not a factor of how much money you have. It's about how you live. This was reinforced later when my sister and I lived together in West Hollywood in a bungalow that we rented for $235 a month. We lived on a dead-end street and knew everyone on our block. We were happy and had a good time.

Father taught us a lot about friendship. He loves to entertain guests and you should hear him sing "Guadalajara." He's actually a terrible singer, but sings that particular song with great gusto! With my mother's excellent cooking, they made entertaining seem very natural. There were times in the early years that she would complain when he brought someone home to dinner unexpectedly. However, my mother became more relaxed as she got older and gradually grew to welcome an unexpected guest with sincere enthusiasm. She'd just set an extra plate on the table for dinner and turn it into a dinner party. Being able to share good food, good conversation and camaraderie became one of her greatest joys, and she passed that gift to all four of her children.

THE CHATTY COOK

Perhaps the easiest way I've found to combine cooking and socializing is an approach I use almost every Sunday. This is the time when I usually cook a big pot of soup or beans. The crucial ingredient is not food, but an inexpensive headphone I bought at an electronics store. (Lots of portable phones are now headset enabled also.) I set everything up with all the veggies washed, the pot on the stove, and the music on the kitchen CD player. I also pour myself a glass of wine. Then, using the headphone, I call one of my girlfriends or family members and talk while I chop. It's quite fun. And before I've even gotten through a half-hour conversation (with some people, that is not a long one), the veggies are all chopped and whatever I'm making is bubbling away on the stove. I consider this basic multitasking. I can do an excellent job of chopping and talking simultaneously.

*"In proceeding to the dining-room,
the gentleman gives one arm to the lady he escorts,
it is unusual to offer both."*

Lewis Carroll

"For me, eating out means laughing, conversing and breaking bread with friends and family. The challenge of staying close to my dietary preferences is a welcome one. "

Chapter Twenty-Two

EATING OUT & TRAVELING

THE RESTAURANT CHALLENGE

Is eating out a hedonistic activity? You probably have an emotional reaction in your answer that reflects how often you eat out, whether it tends to be for business, practicality or pleasure, and how you feel about it. Is this something you enjoy? Would you rather be at home? Is it, logistically, the easiest way to get the kids fed early in the evening, so they can be in bed by a decent hour?

If you rarely go out to eat, you probably consider it a treat and rightfully think you can "afford" (in terms of the cost to your health) to order whatever you want. On the other hand, if you eat out frequently—either because of your work, or to save the time and energy required to shop, cook and clean up after dinner—the pleasures of restaurant eating can impair your health. For that reason, some insight into how to find the happy medium between health and pleasure in restaurant eating could be useful.

I enjoy eating in restaurants. For me, it means laughing, conversing and breaking bread with friends and family. It's a treat for me, because my husband and I rarely go out all by ourselves.

I also delight in travel, having never had to do too much

of it purely for business. From this perspective, the challenge of finding ways to remain reasonably close to my dietary preferences is a welcome one.

This is not to say that I don't have strong preferences as to where the group chooses to eat. As the percentage of people who are vegetarians is small, I know the meat-eaters among you will wonder why you should bother reading about how a vegetarian finds something suitable at a restaurant.

The reason is this: Even if you're not a vegetarian yourself, you still want to eat well. You might learn that it's possible to eat well and healthily by observing how I would choose. I've become very good at navigating menus in most kinds of restaurants so that I don't have to impose my diet on the rest of the party.

Note: When someone in your party has dietary needs based on health, it's best to be gracious about their needs and requests. If they say, "Can we go someplace else? I can't eat at such and such a restaurant because of my diet," I hope you'll take a deep breath and mentally honor the fact that most individuals with dietary needs feel very uncomfortable about imposing them on a whole group. And it's absolutely true that in some restaurants, there will be nothing on the menu that will work for them.

I've had this same problem in the French Quarter in New Orleans. I couldn't find anything vegetarian on the menu but the side dishes. Yet the music was so great, I didn't care!

The fact that I've been eating successfully as a vegetarian for the past 20 years makes me much more sensitive to the needs of other people who, not by choice but as a condition of their health, have to request the understanding of the group. If you have never experienced such a situation, I expect that, sooner or later, you will.

For example, you'll never see me voting for a barbeque place. It's one of the few types of restaurants where there is nothing on the menu that I can eat except the side dishes, and who wants to make a meal of coleslaw if you go out for dinner? A person who is conscientiously avoiding saturated fats (animal fats) would also have a problem with such a restaurant.

Steak houses are almost in the same category, but they usually serve reasonably good salads or offer a salad bar, as well as baked potatoes. And if it's a decent steak house, the wine should be pretty good. So I can enjoy the meal and survive. A steak house can usually serve a piece of fish grilled, so eating there isn't too much of a hardship for a person watching their weight.

I've eaten enough steamed vegetable plates in "Continental" restaurants to last me the rest of my life. But since the wines and service in those establishments are usually a pleasure, I'm content if there's also a good salad and good bread to make up for a bland collection of overcooked vegetables. Again, they should be able to serve a piece of grilled meat, poultry or fish that accommodates most dietary preferences. Because they usually employ a chef, these restaurants are likely to be able to adapt to an individual's needs and preferences.

I am happiest in an Italian restaurant. I never tire of pasta with a tangy tomato and basil sauce. Italian works well for almost everyone, unless a person just doesn't like this type of food. An exception would be if a person is on a low-carbohydrate diet and there are only pasta dishes on the menu.

In a Mexican restaurant, I have lots of choices. Usually it includes pinto beans (I'm a great fan of this basic food item, and my digestive system has become rather well adapted to them). From my experience, most Mexican restaurants now serve *fajitas* (a dish of grilled chicken or steak with grilled vegetables, served with rice or tortillas). If you choose either a chicken or veggie *fajita*, it's possible to eat well without eating too many saturated fats. This is true as long as you are able to refrain from eating too many chips and guacamole. A Mexican restaurant can usually serve the needs of people with allergies.

There are always lots of wonderful choices in Indian and Asian restaurants for almost any dietary need. Vietnamese restaurants have the most wonderful soups! If the members of your party don't like spicy food, you would more naturally steer toward a Chinese or Japanese restaurant, rather than Indian or Thai.

An important thing to understand is if you're trying to reduce your intake of foods high in saturated fat, spices can more than make up for the loss of flavor you encounter when you subtract fried foods, pork, beef and rich sauces. That's why I find the ethnic restaurants more appealing than Continental restaurants that only have a steamed vegetable plate to offer a vegetarian.

Some people have trouble digesting spicy food. However, I believe it's something that you can develop a tolerance for over time. I know because my husband was the original "chili wimp." I call him C.W. sometimes for that very reason. But now he often surprises me by saying a particular salsa is *too* mild. I try not to over-season food for his sake. I've seen him become so uncomfortable in an Indian restaurant that he was practically turning colors.

This brings up the point that if you have no tolerance or appreciation for spicy food, you should ask for mild foods at ethnic restaurants. They are used to accommodating a variety of tastes and should be able to steer you away from any menu choices that they know will be too spicy. And if the food still arrives too spicy, send it back to the kitchen for them to do over. Sometimes "not spicy" means different things to different people.

It's interesting that the restaurants that work for me also tend to be the ones that work for my sister Lynn. She cannot eat wheat, yeast or anything that has gluten in it, but the ethnic restaurants can accommodate her needs because they're more rice- and corn-based than wheat-based. Between us, my sister and I cover a wide band of the "special eating requirements" spectrum. Where we differ is that I can eat bread, which she can't. On the other hand, she eats meat, which I don't.

I asked a friend who is diabetic and allergic to garlic what she enjoys when eating out. She mentioned a favorite restaurant that serves nicely grilled fish. Ellen also says she would rather dine out less often and go to a better quality restaurant, more skillful at accommodating the parameters of her diet.

I concur. In better restaurants, I've persuaded a chef to "invent" a pasta dish when there were no vegetarian entrees on the menu.

DINING OUT WITHOUT GAINING WEIGHT

Even if you never encounter the challenge of restaurant-eating with anyone who is either severely allergic or a committed vegetarian, there's bound to be someone in your party who's either openly or discreetly trying to watch their weight. In fact, if you've gotten this far in my book, that person striving to enjoy eating sensibly is likely to be you!

If you've been watching your diet for years, this next section may seem like old hat to you. But for readers just starting to make these better choices, a hearty word of encouragement. Persevere. Your tastes will gradually change, especially as you achieve some success in finding acceptable alternatives.

In any eateries but the impossible places (coffee shops, delicatessens and fast food restaurants), a big part of your success depends on skillfully negotiating the time between when you sit down and when you're served your main course. There are certain pitfalls at a restaurant and one of them is bread. One slice of bread won't do you in, but stop there.

My suggestion is to tell the waitress that you're about to faint with hunger. Ask if she can bring you a bowl of broth-based soup or a salad right away—provided you like these foods.

I do. Unless we're eating in an ethnic restaurant where it's not really part of the cuisine, I almost inevitably eat a salad. And I think salads are a lot better now than they were 10 years ago. The growing use of baby greens and tasty alternatives (such as arugula) to iceberg and romaine, plus light vinaigrette dressings instead of heavy mayonnaise-based dressings, have vastly improved the general fare.

But if you're not in an establishment that serves these more European-type salads, you can still avoid excessive fat content without sacrificing taste by asking for the dressing on the side, plus lemon wedges. Squeeze the lemon juice over the greens and dip each fork-full of your salad lightly into the dressing. Or better yet, dip your fork into the dressing and then into the salad! It actually improves the taste of the salad in my opinion because you can taste the greens, instead of being overwhelmed with the taste of the dressing.

It's still a little too often that I'll go into a restaurant and find that every salad will include some form of meat— with prices raised as a result. I'm glad to see this is also changing. I trust you can empathize. A chef's salad isn't much of a salad when you subtract the ham, the turkey and the cheese, and who would feel that they hadn't been short- changed if they had to pay the price of a chef's salad with- out those ingredients?

Occasionally, perhaps when traveling, I find myself again in a 1950s time-warp restaurant that considers iceberg let- tuce with a tomato wedge a salad. That's with French, Thou- sand Island or blue cheese bottled dressing. It makes a pretty pathetic lunch, and if that's the totality of your experience with salads, I understand if you don't like them. When faced with such salads, I resort to French fries. As we know, this is the opposite of a smart-fat food choice, but I do enjoy French fries occasionally.

Any establishment above the level of a fast food restau- rant, a delicatessen or a coffee shop should have meat, chicken or fish that is steamed, poached, broiled, roasted, baked or grilled. They may normally serve that entree with a sauce that dramatically hikes up the saturated fat grams and calorie count, but you should be able to head them off at the pass on that. Just tell them to leave off the sauce.

This won't work, however, if there's nothing on the menu that can be adapted. A friend of mine who works as a chef tells me cooks are paid only about $8-$9 an hour in Los Angeles. It's hard and fast work for that amount of money. Also, many cooks are often only allowed to work part-time, so they don't receive benefits. A person has to qualify as a chef to get a decent hourly rate of pay. You can see why some of the cooks in lower-cost restaurants might not be motivated to work around your dietary preferences.

Fast food? "Have it your way" is just a slogan, and it's a nice one. However, if you're on a specific diet of any kind, you really can't have it your way in any fast food establishment.

Avoiding fast food joints, delicatessens and coffee shops is part of the plan I recommend. If you can safely predict that there's going to be nothing on the menu that works for you, try hard to steer the group toward an alternate spot. Or eat something healthy before you join the group and then just have a beverage with the others. Food is hard to resist when you're hungry, so don't go to an unhealthy place when you're starving.

EATING ON THE ROAD

Let's touch on some of the difficulties that one may encounter while traveling. Personally I'm grateful that Taco Bell is nationwide. I agree that it isn't very authentic Mexican food, but it gives me the assurance that I can find something to eat that doesn't have meat in it. And I can ask them to leave the cheese out of the burrito and it will then be lower in fat as well.

At McDonalds, I used to eat French fries until I found out that beef fat is part of the distinctive flavor of their fries. Their pre-prepared salads don't deserve to be called salads. However, McDonalds has often provided me a clean restroom and a cup of coffee. Since the need for either can cause some urgency, I don't want to seem ungrateful.

The Wendy's and Carl's Jr. fast food chains have salad

bars. Wendy's also sells baked potatoes. If you eat a potato without sour cream and butter, that's a filling, nutritious alternative. What might you eat on it? See what they have behind the counter that might normally be used on burgers. If you're lucky, they might have some salsa or chopped tomatoes. Maybe they could grill some onions for you.

If this is a road trip, a little condiment kit to carry into fast food restaurants could be a big help. It could include smart-oil dressings and soy sauce or Bragg's Amino Acids (unfermented and more healthy than soy sauce, but otherwise rather similar). The Bragg's product is available in small bottles. Your kit could also include olive oil and balsamic vinegar. Buy two of the tiny bottles of olive oil at the store, empty one into your large bottle at home and use the empty bottle for balsamic vinegar. Keep salsa packets left over from meals at Mexican fast food restaurants. Health food stores sell vegetarian "BacoBits," which along with sunflower seeds, can dress up either salads or baked potatoes. You won't be able to bring anything that needs to be refrigerated after opening because it might be unsafe to eat after days of being in the car. However there are a number of things that could be brought along that would ease the difficulties of eating wisely on the road. All of these could be stored in a toiletry kit devoted specifically to the purpose and brought discreetly with you into restaurants.

Protein bars are enormously helpful. The bars fulfill the need for something sweet and satisfying, and they generally provide high-quality protein without too much fat (certainly in comparison to fast food possibilities). Buy a box of your favorites and pack them along with you. It will probably be a lot cheaper than buying what you find along the way, plus you can make sure to have something that works when you need it. Almonds are another possibility.

The way Americans approach travel is changing dramatically. Some people never wish to fly again. I'm not totally comfortable flying, but I also know that statistically the most dangerous part of any air trip is the drive to the airport.

If you decide to fly, I'm happy to say that the meals onboard have become more flexible. The airlines will serve a vegetarian meal if you ask for it in advance, and they sometimes can accommodate dairy-free or gluten-free meals. Nevertheless, the best advice I have for traveling is (again) to carry something with you—such as almonds, peanuts, protein bars or even fruit, if its bulk doesn't add too much to what you're already carrying. That way, neither you, nor any member of your party, will be overly affected if it's not possible to meet dietary preferences.

Airports are probably worse than airplanes in terms of their lack of tasty and nutritious food, and the prices are unfairly high. However, I'm pleased to say that the situation is improving. I'm seeing more food courts in airplane terminals that offer a wider variety of food, including more healthy alternatives. If there's a sit-down restaurant in the terminal, you can often find a salad, a cup of soup or something in the appetizer menu that's healthier and more reasonably priced.

TRAVEL TIPS BEYOND MEALS

Here are more tips for avoiding some of the common stressors that take the fun out of traveling.

Can you have a little talk with yourself beforehand? Can you tell yourself that you're not going to fret and worry because worrying really isn't going to change whatever circumstances you encounter? That worrying may only make your experience worse. This mental adjustment is worth practicing.

There has always been confusion and disorientation involved in traveling. But if you make the choice to go, it makes sense to also make the choice to just put up with the hassles.

Fatigue can really impinge on your enjoyment. When planning a trip, give yourself time to rest in case that's really what you need most. I'll confess that I'm getting better at observing this suggestion myself. My sister has waged a solitary campaign to get us all to enjoy more by doing less. Like most campaigns done with patience and persistence, it's beginning to pay off.

Anything that reduces stress and fatigue while traveling is a major contributor to healthy hedonism. It definitely helps you enjoy the trip, and in terms of recreational travel, that is the whole point! This approach is also helpful with business travel.

Here are some commonsense suggestions for reducing stress while flying.

Leave extra early for the airport. The whole airport experience will be a lot less stressful when you don't have to worry about missing your flight. And now with the tighter security, you've got to plan for more "waiting around" time. If you have an early morning flight and you live a long way from the airport, does it make sense to stay the night before at a hotel, or a friend's house, that's closer to the airport?

Sometimes you know that you're going to have to schlep your luggage around a lot during a trip that will last more than a couple days. If this is the case, make it a point to pack several days ahead of time and then do a practice run of

INSIDER TIP ON AVOIDING JET LAG

Here's a hot tip on how to avoid jet lag. It was given to me by an airline pilot. The secret? *Secure an aisle seat and drink a glass of water every hour and nothing else.* No caffeine, no alcohol and no food. All the water will alleviate dehydration, which is one of the problems. The fasting also helps to reset your circadian clock by erasing some of the clues your body uses to tell what time it is. Granted, this approach would be tough to maintain on a marathon overseas flight, one of those 12- to 14-hour ones.

carrying the luggage down the block and back. It may inspire you to start taking a few items out of the suitcase. The sense of mobility gained by having only one small suitcase to lug around, instead of two or three, is a definite contributor to a sense of healthy hedonism while traveling. The travel wardrobes that are becoming available through catalogs (see Resources) can allow you to travel with a fraction of the weight you have carried in the past. It's an investment that you may have to make over a period of time, but just looking at the catalogs can give you ideas of how to begin creating such a wardrobe.

Most people I see at airports nowadays have backpacks or suitcases on wheels. Backpacks distribute weight much more evenly than carrying a suitcase, and that makes the weight feel like much less. The suitcases with wheels also help to make it easier to deal with the weight of what you pack.

Here's another approach you can try: Send a box of clothes ahead of you via UPS or the mail. If you're going to stay with relatives who you visit with some frequency, and at the same times of the year, pick out some nonessentials from your wardrobe and store the clothes at their place. You can wear the same things next time. If they're your family, they shouldn't complain too much about having to store a box of your clothes so you can get through the lines at the airport more quickly. Or they could just ship the box back to you after the trip.

Travel is one of life's most enjoyable experiences. But it's strenuous and that can cause fatigue that greatly affects the pleasure you can derive from your trip. So pace yourself as much as possible.

Finally, it's much easier to change your attitude than to change the circumstances you will encounter while traveling. Like the saying advises, "When in Rome, do as the Romans do."

TIPS FOR TRAVEL BY BUS OR TRAIN

- Bring a pillow and a small, lightweight blanket or a cape you can wrap up in.
- Pack some food. Airports are bad but vending machines are even worse.
- Dress in comfortable clothing, such as sweats.
- Bring earplugs. Crying babies and overly loud talkers can really be an annoyance.
- Don't plan much for the day you arrive. If you've had to spend the night on the bus or train, you're not going to be energetic when you arrive.
- This is a good opportunity to get some reading done. Take along that book you haven't had time to read.
- With any luck, there won't be anyone in the seat next to you. If that's the case, you can stretch out a bit and sleep. The seats are more spacious on busses and trains than on airplanes. This is a good thing, since you usually have to sit in them a lot longer.
- Don't wander too far off when the bus stops for meals. The driver will leave you behind if you don't return to the bus on time.
- Taking the bus or train offers rare people-watching opportunities. Enjoy the variety of people who come into view.

"Enjoyment of special occasions springs from what you bring—literally and figuratively—to a party. Much of that comes from knowing one's self."

Chapter Twenty-Three

MAXIMUM FUN, MINIMAL DAMAGE

WHAT'S YOUR PLEASURE?

A special occasion is a burst of life with the opportunity to enjoy many sensual pleasures before, during and, optimistically, after. When an occasion comes up, we want to be able to relax and enjoy it. But we also want to enjoy the next day and the memories we've created.

Such an occasion should be regarded as far more than an invitation to passively consume. Your enjoyment will have a lot to do with how you prepare, what you bring—literally and figuratively—to a party or event. Much of that comes from knowing one's self. What is it that you want to experience? What will give you the greatest joy? Then really focus on that one aspect of the occasion, and be moderate about the rest of the "banquet."

If I'm truly excited about a concert or show, I often choose to eat lightly and drink only coffee and water throughout the evening. This comes as a reaction to falling asleep during the last act of some world-class ballets.

If food is the centerpiece, I now make no apologies for eating as much as I can. I'll be back to my usual fare the next day.

And if it's the wine, I hope it's a memorable bottle and

make sure I can enjoy it responsibly.

BEFORE THE EVENT

Do you remember the scene in *Gone with the Wind* when Scarlett is dressing to go to the barbeque and her mammy insists she eat before so she won't make a pig of herself later? There was a lot of wisdom in that scene. Only, as adults, we have to prepare for special events without our mammy's coaching.

If you're going to an event where you're likely to have a drink or two and the food will be cocktail nibbles rather than something you could equate with dinner, *eating some real food before you go* means you won't be drinking on an empty stomach. A protein bar or a smoothie provides real nutrients to prevent alcohol from being absorbed too quickly. Minimally, a few gel caps of flaxseed oil or evening primrose oil (as it comes packaged from the health food store) would also coat your stomach, or how about eating a bit of bread dipped in olive oil?

Alcohol is dehydrating, so you can help prevent a hangover by *starting out well-hydrated*. Make sure you drink plenty of water, the whole recommended daily eight glasses—for two to three days leading up to the event.

Upping your intake of fresh fruits, vegetables and brown rice in the days before an event is a form of mild detox that makes sure your system is running smoothly. This can be as easy as hitting a salad bar or a Chinese restaurant for lunch on the days before the event.

Another way to prepare is to have a *carrot and beet juice* combination to provide lots of antioxidants. If you like spicy foods, add a little ginger, which provides powerful protection for the liver. Ginger is spicy, though, so I emphasize "a little."

A common herb that offers liver protection is *garlic*. If you're worried about smelling like garlic, you can buy odorless garlic capsules at the health food store. A couple of 500 mg. capsules during the day helps provide liver cleansing nutrients. While you're at the store, pick up some *milk thistle extract* or *milk thistle tea*. It's generally considered the most powerful herb for enhancing liver function. Combine the milk thistle tea with any other herb tea for additional flavor. It has practically none by itself. There are now many exquisite herb tea blends in health food stores. Just find one that appeals to you and brew a cup of tea with one bag of it and one bag of milk thistle.

Dandelion tea is another good liver detoxifier and it has more flavor than milk thistle tea. There are also *"detox" teas* that blend a number of ingredients. The Yogi Tea variety has a nice flavor. Developing the habit of drinking any of these on an ongoing basis can be one of the easiest health improvements you can make.

AT THE EVENT

Check your mood as you arrive at the event. I can count on one hand the bad hangovers I've had in the past 20 years. A couple of them followed evenings when I was so exhilarated by events at the time that I didn't think about what I was drinking and in what quantities. In retrospect, the occasions were so memorable that a hangover couldn't dampen how fondly I remember them. But now I know that highly positive emotional states can affect one's judgment as easily as highly negative ones. Just the awareness of your susceptibility at such times may be enough to prevent serious consequences!

Staying hydrated at a festivity is extremely important. If you don't want to water down your beverage, try to squeeze in a glass of water between each drink. Ask the bartender to serve it on ice in a highball glass with a wedge of lime.

At restaurants, I order a bottle of mineral water first thing, and keep it coming. I love Pellegrino. Drinking it doesn't seem therapeutic. The mineral content, especially potassium, help replenish the nutrients depleted by alcohol.

Dancing is a great way to work through the effects of food and alcohol. It also pulls you away from tables where they are being served. In addition, it will inspire others through the spirit you display. If you feel that you don't dance well, discard that notion. Few of us dance well, but we can all enjoy it. If no one will dance with you, you can dance by yourself. So long as you're not dancing on a table, no one will regard it as particularly exhibitionist, just expressive.

It's a matter of common sense, but drinking late into the night can dramatically increase your blood alcohol content at a time when your liver expects to be doing its regular housekeeping activities while you're asleep. If you drink late into the night, the only legally and morally responsible ways to do so are by drinking at home, staying the night wherever you are, assigning a designated driver or going home in a cab. The percentage of people driving with a high blood-alcohol level after midnight is way up. These are folks you don't want to meet by accident. So *quit drinking early*. In this way, even if you drink quite a bit, your liver has time to process it before you go to bed.

Still another strategy to minimize damage is to wisely choose what you drink. Carbonation in mixers, or in sparkling wines and champagne, can cause alcohol to be absorbed more rapidly, so avoid bubbles.

The sugar in sweet drinks also speeds up the rate at which alcohol is absorbed. Not only that, but the sweetness is deceptive and it's easy to consume such drinks too quickly. Punch can be dangerous as you often can't tell from the taste how potent it is. Drink something that you're familiar with.

Your liver can only process the alcohol in one ounce of alcohol (approximately one drink) per hour. If you drink faster than that, you're creating a backlog. It can be especially difficult to *keep track of how much you've had to drink* when a host or waiter keeps filling your glass. Use something like the months of the year to remind yourself how many times your glass has been refilled. After four half-glasses of wine, for example, you would be at "April." You might want to slow down long before you reach June.

Though it's the alcohol in your drink that makes you high, it's other ingredients that can make the next morning painful. These substances are called *"congeners"* and they cause the blood vessels to dilate. They're by-products of the fermentation process and create the distinctive flavors of natural wines, beers and spirits. A clue to the number of congeners is the color of the alcohol. White wine, vodka, gin and tequila have fewer than red wine, port, sherry, bourbon, rum, brandy and scotch. Though relatively clear, champagne also has lots of additives. You may have experienced their effect after drinking inexpensive champagne when you found yourself with an instant headache. In general, more expensive alcohols have fewer impurities. It's an additional rationale for buying the good stuff, and besides, you and your friends deserve it.

Remember not to switch what you're drinking in the middle

of, or especially late into the evening. One thing I learned not to do is switch to Irish coffee after drinking margaritas all evening. Champagne on top of scotch is another no-no, even if it is Dom Perignon! I've survived the decision to open a different kind of wine late at night several times, but last time I tried this, it was a mistake. I'll think twice next time.

Women readers should note that right before, or the first days of a monthly cycle can be a precarious time for over-indulgence. The liver is already working overtime to process extra hormones circulating in the system.

LATER THAT NIGHT

Your inclination when you arrive home from a party may be to just fall into bed. However, if you remember to do even a couple of small things, it can greatly improve how you'll feel the next day.

One is to *take your vitamins*. Double up on the antioxidants (C, E, beta carotene and a multi-mineral tablet) and take a B-complex vitamin. You've created a lot for your liver to work on. Give it something to work with.

Drink several glasses of water. This might mean you'll be getting up in the night to urinate. When you do, drink more water.

Whether or not to take a headache remedy as a preventive measure before bed *is a matter of choice* and personal experience. Tylenol (acetaminophen) is easier on your stomach, but hard on your liver. If you drink a lot or have any history of liver problems, don't use Tylenol.® Aspirin is gentlest on your liver. However, it can be hard on your stomach. And though it is not aspirin, anyone who has had side effects from aspirin or any other pain reliever should not take ibuprofen (Aleve® and Motrin®). Excedrin® is aspirin with caffeine and you don't need caffeine when you're trying to go to sleep. Anyone on medication should not take pain relievers and/or alcohol without checking with a physician.

A short walk helps immensely to clear your head with fresh air and a gentle boost to your circulation system. If you didn't quit partying early in the evening and you don't live in a great neighborhood, you might consider this problematic. An alternative might be to do a little dancing in your kitchen, but be careful not to disturb your neighbors.

THE NEXT MORNING

My favorite way of starting any day is by *eating fruit*. But it can be especially welcome the day after a party. Its clean, cool sweetness is like a welcome rain. If you can buy organic fruit, all the better. Pineapple, grapes and watermelon are particularly beneficial. If it's mid-winter and not much fruit is in season, buy a combination of both fresh and frozen fruits before the party, and make a sort of slurpy juice blend from them. Some say that you should avoid the more acidic citrus fruits, because your stomach may be a bit uneasy. I personally don't find that to be true, but I'm not prone to stomach distress.

This is a great time for *juicing*, lots of it. The nutrients from fresh juice are really beyond compare. Juices supply many of the minerals and electrolytes lost to alcohol.

Continuing to *drink a lot of water* is also important. If you add fresh *lemon*, it can help bring your system back to normal. Lemon juice is a valuable detoxifier.

All of this is assuming that you're not so hungover that nothing will stay down. That's a situation that I find one has to wade through on an hour-to-hour basis. *Ginger tea*

NATURAL WAYS TO PREVENT HANGOVERS

Health food stores have products that can be very helpful for preventing hangovers without side effects. Here are some suggestions published in the October 1999 issue of *Natural Foods Merchandiser*.

• Take one teaspoon of *Bifidobacterium bifidum* in water before bed. This is a natural bacteria that inhabits the bowel. It breaks down and detoxifies the aldehydes that are a by-product of alcohol metabolism. Aldehydes are very dehydrating, as well as being one of the primary causes of hangover symptoms. *Natren's Bifido Factor* is a product name you could ask for, if you don't want to try to remember the name *Bifidobacterium bifidum*.

• Another excellent product that specifically eliminates aldehydes is an Ayurvedic remedy called *Liver Care* or *Liv 52* by Himalaya USA.

• *LiveRx* by Metabolic Response Modifiers (MRM) offers a potent combination of ingredients that are all helpful to the liver's detoxification processes.

• Experts quoted in the article also suggested that another approach is to mix a spoonful of *bentonite clay*, available at the health food store, with water or juice the night before and again the next morning. Taking this before you go out is also a good idea. Clay has the ability to absorb 40 times its weight in impurities. I've tried this several times during detoxes, and though it sounds terrible, it doesn't have much taste. If you drink it down in a gulp, you won't notice the texture, which isn't that bad anyway. Bentonite is also quite inexpensive.

relieves nausea. *Alka Gold*® (Alka Seltzer® without aspirin) can help, or even a teaspoonful of *baking soda in water*. Then you can periodically test the state of your stomach with *soda crackers*. At the point that the crackers will stay down, a *Coca-Cola*® is helpful. I have no idea why it works—something about that particular combination of sugar and caffeine, but it does. Next, try some plain rice or a plain baked potato.

Folk literature is full of recipes on how to overcome a hangover, most based on "the hair of the dog," i.e. alcohol, as a way to overcome a hangover. One drink the next day can stimulate production of the enzyme the liver produces to metabolize alcohol—dehydrogenase. But if you do this more than every couple of years, I think it's a serious indicator of a drinking problem. It's a matter of self-examination.

One of the liver's myriad functions is to produce bile to help with the breakdown of fats. *Staying away from greasy foods* for a day or so is also a way of making it easier for your liver, which will still be wading through some of its backlog.

A bath with lavender essential oil is soothing and calming and can be a good choice. In fact, any of the *detox baths* mentioned in Chapter 16 would be helpful. It's a good time for a *sauna*, but don't overdo it. Unless you have to work, the "day after" is a time for languid luxury.

And then there's the best follow-up remedy of all—*a nap!*

"To take wine into our mouths is to savor a droplet of the river of human history."
Clifton Fadiman

"The goal is to bring variety to your dinner table and find small, yet intense taste experiences. It's the search for something to savor. "

Chapter Twenty-Four

QUALITY NOT QUANTITY

I find one of the best things about being where I am in life is the ability to truly appreciate some aspects of moderate behavior. I don't remember when it began. Being consistently *immoderate* used to seem important. Feeling good is what seems important now.

With it has come new insight into the old phrase— "quality, not quantity." It turns out to be one of the best ways to indulge without damage. Fortunately there are many who have gone before on this path. That's why gourmet shops were created.

Additionally, a "quality over quantity" philosophy can be a tool that makes it easier to hold the line on weight.

WHERE TO SEARCH

If you haven't already discovered this gourmet tool yourself, I suggest you scout areas near your home or work, and the route in between, for specialty food stores. It could be an English tea room, an Italian deli or a Japanese grocery. It could also be a gourmet store. It will probably be small and have a wonderful and knowledgeable proprietor who is happy to make suggestions. Going to the store itself is part of the adventure. So if it's a little bit out of your way, that's okay.

Hopefully it has wonderful smells. When I say that, what immediately comes to mind are the stores in the greater Los Angeles area that specialize in foods of India. These aren't gourmet stores in the conventional sense, but one whiff of the spices and incense inside and I get high. They have all sorts of unusual foods, with fascinating packaging. The Indian stores also sell prepared foods and that means it can be a good place to have lunch, or buy take-home for dinner. Going into one of these shops is like making a quick trip out of the country. The people I've met in Indian shops have all been "veddy, veddy" friendly. It's definitely a different shopping experience from conventional supermarkets.

If you're lucky, you might find several specialty shops to drop in on when you find yourself in different parts of town.

The idea is to bring variety to your dinner table and find small, yet intense taste experiences. It's the search for something to savor.

AN EXAMPLE—WINE

The idea that inspired this chapter was a discussion regarding red wine. If you don't care for wine, don't drink at all, or already understand the joys of good wine, the discussion is nonetheless worthwhile. The concept translates to other food categories. But I'll use wine and my own life as an example.

I recall some times in college when the objective was clearly to get high. We bought wine by the gallon and one jug to the next tasted pretty much the same. It wasn't until I was in my forties when I began drinking chardonnays that the light began to dawn. I realized that as dedicated as I was to bargain-hunting, spending more on wine might be a good idea. What really improved my experience with wines was my sister's studies at a school of theology in Berkeley. Whatever your mental associations with Berkeley, the city's grocery stores do sell high-quality wine at excellent prices.

All of that is background information for my assertion that once you have tasted really good wine, you can never be happy with the cheap stuff again.

It's not just the taste that is so much more satisfying. It's the extraordinary variety. The old cliché about variety being the spice of life holds true. For some reason, most of us become rather set in our ways. Maybe we're too stressed to even think about doing things in different ways, or we'd rather experience what we know we like than take a chance on something new. But with some foods or beverages—such as wine, there is such richness of variation within a single category that you can never exhaust the possibilities in one lifetime.

I think an analogy to music is a good one. With classical music, for example, the more you know about the composer, the context of his/her life, or the musicians and the conductor, the more you enjoy listening. And with favorite pieces, rather than tiring of them, you enjoy the music more each time. Gradually a piece takes on associations with your life. The memories it brings can spin you instantly into a dream world wherever you hear it.

Taste is similar. Food has the power to evoke memories whether it's wine, fruit or even cheese.

EXPLORE & ENJOY

Whatever your favorite food is—whether it's chocolate, cheese, coffee, salads, cookies, pastries or sausages—therein lies your opportunity to become a gourmet. Explore it. Find the best. Analyze it. Discuss it with a fellow aficionado. Perhaps learn to make it. Travel to see where it's made. These are dimensions that make your life rich, regardless of how much money you have.

Part Four

Weekends Just for You

*"A detox weekend at least once a year is like taking your car
in periodically for an oil change and a tune-up."*

Chapter Twenty-Five

DETOX WEEKENDS

In proposing the concept of healthy hedonism, I'm not implying that we should party every weekend. First of all, such a thing is impossible for most of us, because there's so much we need to accomplish in our "spare" time. Nor can excessive partying be considered healthy.

What I do suggest is a detox weekend at least once a year. Conceptually, this is like taking your car in periodically for an oil change and a tune-up. No one argues about whether that benefits your car. A mild detox accomplishes much the same thing. It helps us to keep our physical "motor" running smoothly by removing some of the impurities.

Detox experts seem to agree that once every season is best. Twice a year is okay, but even once a year is a lot better than never! Some practitioners recommend detoxing even more often than four times a year. However, to me, that's beginning to sound like a lifestyle that only makes sense for people who live in a community of like-minded people, such as a yoga school, not individuals with homes, families and a myriad of activities and obligations.

WHAT "DETOX" MEANS

What is detox? Until now, most people believed this

word described something only individuals with a heavy-duty substance abuse problem had to do. That definition is correct, as far as it goes, but it refers to a form of medically supervised detoxification necessitated by an addiction to alcohol, street drugs, painkillers or prescription tranquilizers.

The broader definition of "detox" is a process that happens naturally within the body. It is the combined effect of several of the body's organs and systems working harmoniously to eliminate toxins from the body.

By extension, detox is also what an individual does to encourage the natural processes of detoxification to occur.

What the body considers a toxin can be one of two kinds—"*exotoxins*" (meaning toxins that originate outside the body) or "*endotoxins*" (that come from within.) Exotoxins are also called "*xenobiotics*" meaning "foreign to the body." An exotoxin or xenobiotic could be any one of thousands of household, agricultural and industrial chemicals to which we're exposed in the course of our daily lives.

An endotoxin originates within the body, in the form of bacterial waste products, antibodies, hormones and cellular material whose biochemical components need to be recycled or excreted.

Here's an overview of how the body's organs and systems work together in the detoxification process.

The *liver* is the "star" of the body's detox efforts. It's the body's primary detoxification organ with literally dozens of tasks on its job description. Only a few of them pertain to detoxification. Before it can do its detox tasks, however, the liver needs a supply of several vitamins, minerals and amino acids that become part of the biochemical alchemy necessary to a healthy organism. According to Sidney MacDonald Baker, M.D., author of *Detoxification & Healing: The Key to*

Optimal Health, "Effective detox cannot work well without critical dietary substances."

(The required nutrients are all included in the list of suggested daily vitamins, minerals, herbs and amino acids found in Chapter 17, "A Time of Peace.")

From these nutrients, the liver produces enzymes that perform a complex two-phase process that changes the toxin from a fat-soluble substance to a water-soluble one. Once the toxin becomes water-soluble, it can be excreted via the kidneys and the bowel. *If the correct balance of nutrients is not present, detoxification cannot proceed!* If detoxification cannot proceed, one of two things happens. Either the toxin is stored in the body's fat tissues waiting until the correct balance of nutrients is available or the toxin circulates in the bloodstream as a "free radical," causing damage to other tissues via oxidation. (Biologically speaking, a free radical is not a political refugee, but rather a molecule missing a hydrogen electron. The presence of the free radical sets off a chain-reaction among cells in which a nearby molecule is stripped of one of its electrons. This, in turn, causes that molecule to strip the electron of another molecule, and so on.)

The process of oxidation causes tissues to age at a much faster rate. Much research, and subsequent publicity, has taken place in recent years to determine which foods and supplements are best in slowing or preventing oxidation. As a result, we frequently hear the phrase "antioxidant" used in the marketing of innumerable nutritional products. It describes the various vitamins, minerals and amino acids— including C, E, bioflavinoids, beta carotene, glutathione, selenium and zinc—that the body uses, biochemically, to neutralize free radicals.

You'll find a more extensive explanation of these processes on *www.thehealthyhedonist.com*. Click on "How to Detox," which links to our affiliated website—*www.detox.org*. You can also learn a great deal more by reading *The 20-Day Rejuvenation Diet Program* by Jeffrey Bland, Ph.D., or *The 7-Day Detox Miracle*, by Peter Bennett, N.D., and Stephen Barrie, N.D.

Assisting the liver is the *circulatory system*, which delivers nutrients to every cell in the body via the blood. The heart is the center of this system and it pumps blood out through major blood vessels called arteries. The arteries become smaller and smaller until blood cells move through them single-file. These microscopic blood vessels are called capillaries. They permeate every tissue of the body except hair and fingernails.

At the capillary level, oxygen and other nutrients in the blood cells move through the porous walls of the capillaries and become part of the interstitial fluid that bathes every cell. The cells absorb the nutrients, and at the same time, they give off waste products, such as carbon dioxide. The waste products diffuse out of the cell and into the interstitial fluid. Most of the waste products then proceed through the capillary walls and into the blood cells, which carry them away for excretion by the *lungs*, *kidneys* and *intestines*. (The rest of the waste products are eliminated via the lymph system as previously discussed in Chapter 8.)

The blood flows from the capillaries into the veins, by which it completes its circuit back to the lungs and heart. As part of its circulation throughout the body, blood picks up nutrients as it flows through the lining of the stomach and small intestines. It flows through the liver, where detoxification takes place. It also flows through the kidneys.

The kidneys continuously filter the blood for the waste materials of cell metabolism, delivered by the bloodstream. From the kidneys, waste is excreted through the urinary tract.

The *small intestine* is more an organ of digestion than of excretion. Those components of food, such as fiber, that cannot be digested in the small intestine proceed to the *large intestine*. These leftover food substances can putrefy if they remain too long in the large intestine, which causes toxins to be reabsorbed through the intestine wall where they re-enter the bloodstream.

The intestines also carry away the toxins that the liver neutralized and then excreted into bile. Before reaching the intestines, the bile moves from the liver to the bile duct, and then on through the pancreas.

Although the *lungs* give off a waste product, carbon dioxide, they are not considered part of the excretory system but rather the respiratory system. Our lungs pull oxygen from the air, deliver it to the bloodstream, and then the process is reversed. In the second part of the process, carbon dioxide is pulled from the blood, and the lungs exhale it.

HOW & WHY PEOPLE DELIBERATELY DETOX

The purpose of a deliberate detox is to encourage all these processes to happen more efficiently. The work of the natural detoxification system can be enhanced by a few changes in our behaviors on a short-term basis, such as during a detox weekend. These changes include the following:

1. *Avoiding the food that you normally eat,* so your body can work on cleansing itself, instead of carrying out its normal digestion and metabolic processes.

2. *Increasing the intake of substances that naturally cleanse the body*. These include water and fresh fruit and vegetables, or juices made from them. The water, fruit, vegetables and juices are high in the nutrients essential to detoxification. On this list are also herbs that promote a cleansing effect. I'll say more about these toward the end of this chapter.

3. *Resting*, so that your body can perform the cleansing functions, instead of the biochemical activities required in moving around.

In short, a detox can be regarded as a spring cleaning for your body, regardless of when you do it. Similar to an intensive period of housecleaning once a year, it's about providing the time and nutrients for the body to concentrate on these activities instead of the processes you normally ask it to perform. The benefits that most people describe are those of feeling "lighter" and more energized and clear-headed. Another result that people often mention is feeling more optimistic. Weight loss can be an additional benefit, but to approach detox only for the sake of weight loss is to miss many of the lessons the process has to teach.

Why do we need to detox if this is a natural process? The two-word answer is simple—toxin overload. Our bodies are equipped to handle the endotoxins mentioned earlier, not all the exotoxins of the 21st century.

Our environment contains thousands of toxic chemicals. While we may attempt to dodge them, there are many that are difficult, if not impossible to avoid. For example, many of us live in places where the air and water are anything but pristine. Yes, we have the option to move, but can we earn a living in a place that's less polluted? The issues around how to avoid toxins become very complex.

Very few of us are able to eat a "pure" diet. We are ingesting residual chemicals from pesticides, herbicides and fertilizers in our produce. And as for meat and dairy products, I suggest you read *Mad Cowboy* by Howard Lyman.

Even when we make efforts to avoid toxins, the truth is that our bodies are being exposed to levels that have never been present before. We know the Romans were exposed to lead via their plumbing. We know the air pollution from the factories of 19th century England was sometimes fatal. But the magnitude of the chemical "soup" in which we live was never present before the last half of the 20th century and, certainly, there have never been the variety of sources we experience today. Conventional building techniques, furniture made from plywood and other composite "presswood" materials, clothing, toys, office equipment and automobiles all "outgas" the chemicals that were used to make them. Our choices in personal care products, laundry products and what we choose as our indulgences also add to our body's chemical load. Last, but not least, are emotional toxins. Negative emotional states create stress hormones that our liver has to process along with all the toxins.

For more detailed information regarding chemical exposure and how to find ways to reduce it, see the website *www.thehealthyhedonist.com* and click through to the affiliated website *www.detox.org*.

I don't present this list to scare you. The good news is that with detox weekends, there is something you can do about it. Will it totally remove the threat that chemicals pose to your health? No, but it can *reduce* the danger they pose, especially if, as you become increasingly aware, you take action to avoid superfluous toxins. (It's a free country and you are allowed to decide which ones those are.)

There are no guarantees in terms of health, but if you take responsibility, become increasingly better informed, and cautiously experiment (based on your own educational efforts and the advice of a licensed, holistically oriented practitioner), detoxification can be a powerfully effective way to protect and improve your well-being.

A CAUTIONARY NOTE

There are some people who should not detox without the supervision of a licensed medical practitioner experienced in detoxification. Such people include children, pregnant or nursing mothers, anyone who is taking medication or is suffering from a serious and debilitating illness, and anyone who has been exposed to high levels of very toxic materials.

To find an appropriate healthcare practitioner near you, see the "Finding Allies" section of our affiliated website *www.detox.org*. Contact information for several organizations and clinics is also listed in the Resources for Chapters 25 and 28 at the back of the book.

PREPARING FOR A DETOX WEEKEND

CAFFEINE REDUCTION

I strongly suggest you taper down on how much caffeine you drink during the week before you first try detoxing.

Otherwise you're quite likely to experience a terrible caffeine withdrawal headache. Just remember, a lot of carbonated drinks also contain caffeine.

I've switched my approach to caffeine over the past year to drinking organic green tea in the morning. Green tea has less caffeine than coffee, and it also has significant levels of antioxidants. The tea is best when it has been freshly brewed. (Green tea becomes bitter when it's overbrewed or cold.) I won't say that I'm wild about the taste of green tea, but gradually I've become fonder of it. There are many varieties of flavored green teas available if the taste of one type isn't to your liking.

Though green tea is not *generally* recommended, some detox books allow it during detox. (None allow coffee.) If you have a real caffeine dependency, green tea provides a mild hit—enough to keep you from going into withdrawal. It's a compromise in terms of detox because green tea is high in antioxidants and definitely provides nutritional benefits.

I certainly believe that drinking green tea during your detox is better, long term, than feeling so horrible from a caffeine withdrawal headache that you can't function and never want to voluntarily go through a similar experience again. In general, drinking green tea is a good habit to cultivate.

I still indulge in a cup of coffee or two in the afternoons on most regular days. By most healthcare guidelines, this is still too much caffeine. But hey, if I were perfect, I would be writing a different book!

WHEAT AND DAIRY REDUCTION

If you eat a lot of wheat and dairy, it's also good to taper way down on them during the week leading up to your detox.

That way, your system will have time to adjust more gradually to the change in diet. What would you substitute? Well, rice for one. The good news is that you can find rice in many forms at the health food store that you can't find at a supermarket. You can find rice cereals, rice bread and even rice pastas. In fact, if you ask the personnel at the health food store, they will be able to suggest many substitutes for wheat and dairy products. It's a good idea to also transition out of the detox weekend with rice products, instead of going back to your old favorites immediately. Of course, if you've found the substitutes to be reasonably pleasant, consider sticking with them for a longer time to see if you can make a more permanent shift in your diet.

BOWEL REGULARITY

If you're not regular, and that means at least one bowel movement a day, you might want to work on regaining regularity before you do a detox weekend. It's like cleaning the leaves out of the rain gutters before the rainy season begins.

Colonics and enemas can help with this aspect. If this idea is offensive to you, then take another approach. Herbal bowel cleansing kits, often referred to as "detox" kits, are available at health food stores. They have been known to improve regularity for many people and you might be one of them. (While I believe the products have great benefit in terms of bowel cleansing, which is an important step in detoxification, herbal bowel cleansing is only one of a number of ways to eliminate toxins from your body. Also, the instructions that come with these kits are not an adequate medium to educate a consumer regarding detox. But as long as you understand that these products do not represent a comprehensive approach to the large subject of detox, you won't be confused.)

These products are formulated with a number of different herbs. Some of them, such as cascara sagrada (*Rhamnus purshiana*) and senna (*Cassia acutifolia*), have a strong laxative effect. They also include herbs, such as milk thistle (*Silybum marianum*), that support the liver and enhance its detoxification processes. If you use one of these products, follow the instructions carefully and observe your reactions. I once experienced strong emotional reactions to taking an herbal detox product, which I think was caused by rapid detoxification of hormones.

If you're not quite ready to take the suggestions I've offered in the last two paragraphs, drinking eight glasses of water and a serving of brown rice each day should improve your regularity. All whole grains have fiber, but brown rice is better than others because of its ability to absorb toxins as it passes through the intestines.

If you do this and find you're not experiencing any gastrointestinal distress from the brown rice, you can even do a *brown rice fast* in which you eat only brown rice for a day or two. This is one of the easiest forms of fasts to do initially because it's more "mechanical" than "biochemical." An organic brown rice fast simultaneously expedites the excretory process and detoxifies the large intestine. It's a simple fast (but do buy *organic* brown rice). You don't have to worry about being hungry or getting the jitters. It's just a little boring. I suggest seasoning the rice with Bragg's™ Amino Acids, available at all health food stores. This Bragg's product has a similar taste to soy sauce but is much better for you because it isn't fermented and has only naturally occurring sodium. A fail-safe recipe for cooking brown rice is included in Recipes at the back of this book. Be sure to drink lots of water during the brown rice fast.

Another way to improve regularity is to add a tablespoon of ground flaxseed to your morning cereal or smoothie. Eating a couple of apples a day is also excellent because they have apple pectin, a water-soluble fiber that absorbs cholesterol, reduces blood sugar imbalances, and is mildly detoxifying. A couple of glasses of juice a day with a teaspoon of psyllium husk or apple pectin (both available from health food stores) is another way to add fiber. Always follow such a fiber drink with a glass of water. Eating high fiber cereals, such as oatmeal or All Bran,® is still another way to promote regularity.

If you have *chronic* constipation, rather than using an herbal kit, I strongly urge you to consult with a licensed holistically oriented healthcare professional. Chronic constipation is a clear indication that you need to make some changes to your diet. Plus you'll feel much better if you can stay regular without using over-the-counter laxatives, on which you can become dependent.

THE WEEKEND DETOX

Many of the recent books on detox suggest rather long processes lasting a week, 10 days, or even longer. I believe, however, that a detox of that length is something one must work up to doing. You may want to eventually plan a longer detox, but right now I suggest that you begin with just a weekend.

How do you conduct a detox weekend? There are lots of detoxification methods, but I have found that one good approach is a *fresh fruit and vegetable fast*.

True fasting means drinking only water. Why not just

do a water fast? Well, a water fast will bring on rapid detoxi-fication. You might have reactions that are unpleasant, such as headaches, nausea, feelings of emotional uneasiness and light-headedness. Rapid detoxification can be more than unpleasant. It can be dangerous. It causes high levels of tox-ins stored in fatty tissues to be released into the bloodstream. You may have experienced this in a small way as the jitters you feel when dieting. At high levels, those toxins can cause oxidative stress to other tissues unless you have the right combination of nutrients circulating in your bloodstream. Oxidative stress ages tissues. That happens fast enough, so why speed up the process by being overly ambitious in an effort to improve your heath?

In the case of a fruit and vegetable fast, I use the word "fast" to mean that you restrict your food intake for two or three days to only fruits and vegetables. Within those pa-rameters, you have many options, depending on your pref-erences and the season. I also strongly urge you to use cer-tified organic produce.

Most people prefer fruit in the morning and vegetables in the evening. You can eat the vegetables raw in a salad, juiced, steamed or cooked into a soup. (See Recipes in the back of this book.) Another approach is to do a *"mono-fast."* This means eating only one kind of fruit for a couple of days. Good choices would be either watermelon or grapes. You could do it with almost any kind of fruit that isn't too acidic, meaning plums or citrus are not a good choice. A mono-fast is a good idea for what to do if your fruit tree produces more bounty than you can otherwise eat or pre-serve.

The quantity of fruit and vegetables you eat during the weekend is up to you. I would probably eat about one piece of fruit every hour in the morning, then have a big salad for lunch. I'd have more fruit and freshly squeezed juice in the afternoon. And then I'd have some soup or steamed veggies for dinner and go to bed early. You don't have to be hungry during the detox weekend. Eating during this special weekend is not only the means of detoxing, but a central part of the entertainment. So buy wonderful fruit and savor it. Make an incredible salad and enjoy it. Be extravagant in your implementation. A sense of deprivation is to be avoided.

Juice fasting is frequently recommended in books on the subject of detox. However, I don't suggest you go that route if you've never tried any sort of detox procedure before. This is because juice fasting, all by itself, is a very fast way of detoxing, and it also promotes rapid weight loss. It seems that a lot of models and celebrities are using this means to lose weight before fashion shows or events. Because a juice fast means no solid food, and because you then recommence eating a lot of food compared to how much you were eating during the fast, there's a purge/binge dynamic here that's unhealthy. More than three days of a liquid fast is an extreme form of detox. The speed of the detoxification can bring on very unpleasant reactions.

As herbalist C. J. Poutinen says in her book, *Herbs for Detoxification*, "People who are young, healthy, active, health-conscious, well-nourished and free from major toxins can embark on the most arduous cleansing programs with good results and few side effects, but for most of us, ambitious programs are best approached with caution and common sense." She goes on to explain that because it is possible for most people to get rid of stored toxins without unpleasant side effects, it doesn't make much sense to approach the project in a way that has a very high probability of causing those reactions.

This is not to say that I'm against juicing. I think juicing is great. It's delicious. It's nutritious. And it's fun to try out different combinations. Fresh juices not only can, but should be combined with a couple of days of eating whole fruits and vegetables. They're marvelous as between meal snacks and pick-me-ups, whether you're detoxing or not.

If you do find yourself feeling a bit funky while doing either fruit-juice or whole-fruit fasting, remember one simple rule. Fruit speeds up the detox, vegetables slow it down. So eat more vegetables if you find you're feeling just a bit worse than you want to feel. If you feel really lousy, eat a small amount of plain white rice. This will slow the detoxification process considerably. As soon as you feel better, you can resume your fasting regime.

An important aspect of detoxing is rest. This is not the time to have a garage sale, much less run a marathon or even do a great number of errands. It might be a good day to go to the gym, not to work out but to take a sauna. (I'll say more about that in Chapter 28, "Spa Culture without Big Bucks.")

I plan my detox weekends around really low-key activities, such as catching up on movies I've missed. At the same time, I whittle down my accumulation of mending. Reading, napping and bathing are also good choices. I eliminate social events. The next three chapters include information on other activities that can be added to this light fasting format.

LEARNING ABOUT DETOXING

Lots of reading and experimentation is the answer to learning more about detox. I learned by a gradual switch away from meat, poultry, fish and dairy. This was detoxifying in itself. Later, at a time when I pursued yoga more intensively, I began to try fasting. That's when I found out how caffeine withdrawal can affect you during a fast. Watermelon fasting was my favorite approach at that time.

Since then, information on detox has exploded, and we now see the subject of detoxification bursting into the mainstream media with articles in the *Los Angeles Times* and the *USA Today* "Weekend" supplement.

As I read most of the books available, I did another level of experimentation with detoxing. I quickly began to feel major cumulative effects. Finally, in the past two years, I dramatically increased the amount of exercise I've been getting, as well as the number of supplements I take. I've switched to eating more protein and eating it earlier in the day. And also, because I now work from home, I'm able to get a little more sleep than I did when I worked in an office every day. As a result of these changes, I have more energy now than 15 years ago. I can tell you from personal experience that all of this can work, but I also urge you to go at it with a sense of adventure and exploration. We all come with the same parts, but we're highly individual. With persistence, you will discover what's best for you personally.

As I mentioned before, there are many ways to detoxify. For that reason, don't be confused by what might seem to be conflicting information. Finding what works for *you* is what's important.

One source of confusion can come from skeptics, including physicians, who say that there's no need to detox because the body does it naturally. This, I think, fails to take into account how big a problem toxicity has become in this country. Cancer rates are an obvious indicator. Watching the relative rates at which people age is another. Ask yourself why some people are peppy and energetic at 50, while others have become middle-aged? It isn't just genetics. In general, the well-known recommendations for good health—such as exercising, taking vitamins, eating fruits and vegetables and reducing stress—can be seen as important elements of a comprehensive approach to promoting the body's natural detoxification processes on a day-to-day basis. Detoxification prevents the oxidative stress to tissue throughout the body that manifests as aging.

DETOX SUPPLEMENTS

In recent years, herbal medicine has reemerged as a respected healing modality. The following section describes herbs that can enhance your body's natural detoxification processes. These can be used not only during a detox weekend, but also on a regular basis. The herbs I'm listing below have been used reliably by herbalists and naturopathic physicians for a long time.

With all herbal supplements, unless you're under the supervision of a *licensed* holistically-oriented practitioner and following his/her recommendations, it's good to begin with a small amount of just one substance at a time and gradually build up to a larger amount. That way, if you have an allergic reaction, for example, you know what you're reacting to. It's also possible that a reaction such as mild headache or slight nausea shows the herbs are working to bring toxins back into the bloodstream from storage in fat tissue. That's good, but the feelings are not pleasant. Cut back the amount and see how it makes you feel. If you still feel unpleasant, try another herb and see how that works for you.

There are several ways to take these herbs. You might

take one as a detox tea several times a week, gradually increasing to every day. You could also add a capsule of milk thistle, for example, to your daily selection of vitamins and minerals. Or you can add a fluid herbal extract to a smoothie or to a flavored herbal tea. In any case, buy a good brand from a major health food store so you're sure the herbs are fresh. The owner or manager can help you to find a reputable brand. Then follow the package instructions carefully.

Milk thistle (Silybum marianun) is at the top of the detox supplement list. This herb has been scientifically researched in Europe for more than 45 years and has no known toxicity. Milk thistle is a powerful antioxidant that protects the liver, promotes the flow of bile, and acts as a general tonic to a number of other organs. It stimulates the creation of new liver cells.

Milk thistle's effectiveness against toxins has been documented through its use as an antidote to, among other substances, poisonous mushrooms. It has been used to treat numerous liver diseases. (If for some reason you think you might have a liver disease, don't self-treat. See a *licensed* holistically-oriented healthcare practitioner immediately.)

This herb also helps prevent depletion of the amino acid glutathione in liver cells. Glutathione is one of the nutrients essential to the detoxification process.

Milk thistle is commonly used as a liquid extract, as a powder in capsules, or as a tea. Between 300 to 600 mg. per day is recommended. Correlate this to the instructions on the packaging. Milk thistle has practically no taste and it can be combined nicely with any tea. I recommend brewing it with green tea to create a highly nutritious, stimulating beverage.

Garlic (Allium sativum) is extremely beneficial to your

health. It enhances the immune system through its anti-bacterial, anti-fungal, anti-viral, anti-candida and anti-parasitic effects.

This bulbous herb aids the circulatory system by lowering cholesterol and fat levels as well as thinning the blood.

In addition to stimulating and protecting the liver, garlic is effective in reversing the effects of lead poisons and hydrocarbons. Garlic helps protect against cancer too. Historically it was used in folk medicine to ward off vampires and for protection from black magic!

Whether or not it is toxic to vampires, garlic has no known toxicity to humans. The Italians have put it thoroughly to the test! In addition to eating garlic in food, one can buy capsules of odorless garlic. A suggested dose is 400 mg. a day of a standardized extract.

Burdock root (*Arctium lappa*) is commonly sold in health food stores as a tea. It is both a tonic and diuretic. Burdock helps to remove impurities from the blood, and it aids in restoring efficient liver, gallbladder and kidney function.

This herb is known to stimulate the immune system through its anti-bacterial and anti-fungal properties. It is considered particularly effective in clearing skin diseases, which are often a symptom of toxicity. Burdock is also recommended for gout.

Since burdock can interfere with iron absorption, a person who is anemic should choose another herb.

As a tea, burdock is mildly flavored, with slightly more flavor than milk thistle.

Dandelion (*Taraxacum officinale*): What most people regard as a common weed is a powerful liver tonic, a diuretic, and one of the most effective blood cleansers. Dandelion lowers cholesterol and improves the functioning of the stomach, spleen, pancreas and kidneys.

It's said that dandelion aids in the prevention of both breast cancer and age spots.

And as a tea, dandelion has a very pleasant, slightly nutty taste. All in all, this is something you should add to your repertoire.

Yellow dock root (*Rumex crispus*), also called curly dock and sad dock, is a blood purifier and cleanser. It improves both colon and liver function. In addition, yellow dock is good for anemia, the gall bladder and the spleen. This herb is used in treatment of many skin disorders, especially when combined with sarsaparilla (*Smilax ornata*).

Yellow dock herb is often used as an ingredient in detox and fasting teas.

Red clover (*Trifolium pratense*) is an effective anti-bacterial herb. It is also a blood purifier, an appetite suppressant, and a relaxant.

Red clover is very good to take while healing, and it can be helpful for those with fragile constitutions, including the elderly and children.

This herb is also good for coughs, as it is respiratory specific.

Echinacea (*Echinacea angustifolia*) has become widely known as an herb that stimulates the activity of immune cells that destroy bacteria, viruses and other infectious agents. It is also an excellent lymph cleanser, which makes it valuable as a detoxifier.

Echinacea is nontoxic, and the herb can be widely found in capsule or tablet form in health food and drugstores. It's available as a tea or liquid extract in health food stores. Follow package instructions for use.

Fresh lemon juice is a good liver cleanser. Just add it to water.

This list does not name all the herbs that can facilitate the body's detoxification processes. To do justice to them would require another book, but there's plenty here with which to begin.

I will certainly look forward to hearing back from you (janet@thehealthyhedonist.com) to learn about your experiences with detox. I believe this is a body of information that anyone who is seriously interested in protecting their health should become better acquainted with. As individuals find out how effective detox is in terms of reinforcing their health, reversing chronic conditions and slowing aging, the ripple effect through the healthcare community will be interesting to observe. As Jeffrey Bland, Ph.D., founder of HealthComm International, Inc. (the leading privately funded research company involved in human nutrition), has commented, with this information "you are your own best health insurance provider."

"Depend upon it that, rude and careless as I am, I would fain practice the yoga faithfully."

Henry David Thoreau

"I leave an hour and a half yoga class feeling like I've just returned from a two-week vacation."

Chapter Twenty-Six

YOGA & T'AI CHI

Over the past 30 years, acupuncture has overcome skepticism to become a respected form of alternative medicine. This system of treatment uses very thin needles that are inserted into the body's meridian, or energy, channels. Its success validates this Eastern concept of vital life energy flowing along 12 major pathways of the body.

The good news is that you don't have to find an acupuncturist to get your lifeforce energy flowing more efficiently. Yoga is one very effective way to loosen up any blockages. The buzz one feels after a yoga class is the effect of releasing *prana*, another term for life energy, that had previously been obstructed.

AN INTRODUCTION TO YOGA

In much the same way that acupuncture has been accepted, mainstream society is opening up to yoga. The April 2001 *Time* magazine cover story on the subject reported that 15 million Americans—twice as many as five years previous—now embrace this practice that began in India around 5,000 years ago.

But yoga promises to have an even wider effect than acupuncture, because it can be done by anyone with the

MAY THE LIFE FORCE BE WITH YOU

Westerners are increasingly familiar with the Oriental concept that what we call "life" in a living organism is the outward manifestation of vital energy or life force. Though quite naturally known by different names in the different cultures—*chi* to the Chinese, *ki* to the Japanese, and *prana* in India—the concept is the same. It states that life, energy, enthusiasm, *joie de vivre* (or whatever you want to call it) is an expression of this vital energy that flows through channels called meridians. These channels correspond generally to the primary pathways of the central nervous system.

curiosity to learn it. If you doubt that statement, because you conceive of yoga as a physical skill requiring one to bend one's body into odd positions, I hope to persuade you that one of the beauties of yoga is that it meets you where you are. Because it is a system that uses concentration and breath, in addition to gentle stretching, it can be of great benefit, even to those who are very stiff. What it teaches is a time-honored approach to relaxation, pain relief and stress management, as well as a way to gradually achieve greater flexibility and strength, regardless of one's current physical condition.

Yoga's effects are paradoxical. This practice does energize and tone the body. Yet it achieves this through gentle stretching and rhythmic breathing exercises. Yoga cannot in any way be compared with Western approaches to fitness, such as aerobic exercise or weight training.

Yoga works on an entirely different model. It achieves much of its benefit by releasing tension stored in the muscles. If not released, that tension leads to stiffness. Yoga also teaches you how to quiet the mind, let go of stress, and completely relax. I leave a yoga class feeling like a warm jellyfish with a good sense of energy. The state of well-being that I achieve in an hour and a half is better in terms of effect than most two-week vacations! A good yoga class shouldn't cost you more than $10. In a package deal, it can be even less.

Some skeptics say there is no scientific evidence to support any of the claims of yoga devotees. However, the longevity of the practice, combined with its diverse set of practitioners—including athletes, actors, dancers, New Age seekers and 5,000 years of Indian spiritual masters—seems to indicate it has something to offer.

Devakanya G. Parnell, Director of Resident Yoga Education at the Kripalu Center in Lenox, Masssachusetts, provided the following remark for an article in the *1997 Guide to Yoga Teachers & Classes*. It summarizes the power of yoga. "Within the body is a subtle flow of rhythmic energy pulsations. Even the most insignificant thought can disturb or block this flow. But as you dissolve mental and emotional disturbance through [yoga] practice, tremendous amounts of prana (life force) are released. That life energy spontaneously retards the aging process; it strengthens and rejuvenates all the systems of the body. Thus you progressively accelerate those internal healing processes that enable you to awaken to the higher centers of consciousness."

Thinking of yoga as an energy "tonic" or "tune-up" starts to bring it into a Western perspective. Undoubtedly, yoga has a tangible effect on the nervous system.

Yoga is not a religion. It doesn't proselytize. It begins with stretching, strengthening, energizing and relaxing the body. The yoga student then uses techniques to calm the mind. It can help to heal.

What most of us understand to be yoga is actually a series of techniques, referred to as hatha yoga, developed to loosen and strengthen the body for meditation practice.

GUIDELINES FOR STUDYING YOGA

How might you experience the effects yourself? First, prioritize your goals in attending yoga classes. Are you most interested in strength and flexibility, are you looking for stress management, or are you trying to make new progress in recovering from an old injury? When you know what you want to achieve, I recommend that you look in the Yellow Pages under yoga to find a yoga school or go to *www.yogajournal.com*. (Other websites are listed in Resources.) When you telephone a school, ask if it offers a beginner's class and whether the person teaching the class has been certified. Then ask how long that person has been practicing and teaching. If the teacher has not been certified, if he/she has not been practicing yoga for at least five years, and if he/she has less than two years of teaching experience, look further.

Many yoga schools offer a free initial class. Many have occasional free open houses. These would be additional questions to ask when you telephone the schools.

When you find a school with an experienced teacher, ask if it's possible to speak with the teacher by telephone before you come to the class. That way you could discuss your goals privately with the instructor and get a better understanding of how the class will fit within your goals. The instructor might suggest another place or instructor who might be more in line with what you're trying to accomplish.

You'll need to use discernment in finding an appropriate teacher in the same way that you would use discernment about an art or music instructor's skills. Yoga is not something an instructor can learn to teach during a weekend seminar. To master its subtleties requires intense work with knowledgeable teachers. This is a tradition that is passed from teacher to student who, after years of practice, might eventually become a teacher too. Though videos are a good way to practice at home, and yoga classes at a gym are inexpensive and convenient, the way to learn yoga is to take classes from someone who *knows* yoga and who can guide and gently correct you. That is something you can't experience from a video.

Over a period of time that varies depending on how intensely one practices, yoga can provide an almost miraculous improvement in strength, flexibility and even mental outlook. But the changes in flexibility are not something to be forced. When people try to push themselves into levels beyond their true limits, injuries often result. Several articles have appeared recently reporting a rise in injuries among yoga students.

Because of the growing popularity of yoga, many health clubs now offer it. Major problems can come from taking yoga at the gym, and though I'm not saying that those problems can't happen at a yoga school, they are less likely to happen in a place where the instructor has been sufficiently trained. Yoga's rapid growth in popularity means there aren't enough experienced instructors to meet the demand. One problem that a gym tends to magnify rather than minimize is the competitive spirit of Westerners, who often want to excel at everything they do. Yoga is not a competition, and a good instructor should discourage that attitude. A good instructor will carefully watch newer students and will gently suggest to students how to achieve the benefit of the posture without risk of injury. Some traditions, especially Iyengar Yoga, use props such as straps, blankets and wooden blocks to help those who are less flexible (as we get older, that becomes an increasingly larger percentage of us) to achieve good alignment in the postures. The benefit comes from the correct alignment, not from how far into the posture you can go. That's why it can benefit you regardless of your level of flexibility.

Another mark of a good instructor will be his or her inquiry into a new student's weaknesses and prior injuries. An experienced instructor will be able to show you how to achieve benefit without any danger of aggravating an existing condition. If you are particularly inflexible, have back problems, if parts of your body are significantly weak, or if you have old injuries that still affect you, you need specialized instruction. If the instructor doesn't ask you about your physical limitations, it means the instructor isn't conducting the class with a strong awareness that students come to yoga with varying needs and abilities.

If you find yourself in a class in which the instructor doesn't ask about new students' possible limitations, be careful and conservative in how you attempt to follow the instructions. If a certain pose begins to hurt, back off on the pose immediately. And look for an instructor who can be more attentive to your individual needs.

My last comment about why it's better to study yoga at a yoga school than at a gym is because of the "vibes." This is not something you have to take my word on. Yoga works on a lot of levels. But you won't be able to tap into many of those levels if the class is held in a place where, just outside the door of the yoga class, people are pumping iron and listening to disco, rap or rock 'n' roll. A yoga school collects a cumulative vibration. It is a place of peace. But that vibration can't accumulate in a place that isn't clean, serene and quiet. Try a class in both places. You'll easily notice the difference.

What might you expect in a typical yoga class? One by one, the postures of a yoga routine address the various parts of the body where we accumulate tension.

An hour and a half class at a yoga school would begin with a few breathing exercises, eye stretches, then shoulder and neck stretches. Gradually the class warms up and proceeds to more vigorous stretches, including the Sun Salutation—a series of 12 different poses that flow from one into another. There are the inverted postures—head stands and shoulder stands, though a head stand is rarely part of beginning classes. If it is, don't attempt it prematurely, as it can take months to learn to do them without risk of injury. Forward bends, back bends, spinal twists and balance postures complete the routine, and the class ends with a final relaxation in which the students gently breathe lying flat on their backs, arms and legs relaxed at their side. The lights are dimmed. Though it only lasts a matter of minutes, final relaxation is a profound experience that shows how relaxed you can become.

The poses work to gently stretch various parts of the body. In each, the individual focuses on a point of tension and then breathes into that spot. While exhaling, you let go of tension. You actually blow it right out of your body.

If going to a yoga school seems too strange for you to

do on your own, talk your spouse or a friend into going to a class with you. Wear loose and comfortable clothing. You will probably be asked to remove your shoes at the door. During a yoga school open house is a great time to go for the first visit because the emphasis is completely on welcoming those who have never been there before.

Yoga schools can be a place to meet people who are also searching for meaning and tranquility in a world where solace is rare. And many schools offer vegetarian cooking classes.

Though not a huge danger, I would add one other cautionary note. The major yoga traditions that came to the U.S. from India in the early to mid-20th century are well-established. (See Resources.) They charge reasonable amounts for their classes, seminars and retreats. Since then, there have been a lot of spin-offs. If you find yourself in a yoga school with a lot of emphasis on a charismatic "guru" who charges a lot or pressures you for donations of large sums of money, or anything else, then you're in the wrong yoga school. (I'm happy to say I've never come across this situation, but I hear it happens. Be aware. I want you to have a good experience.)

T'AI CHI—ANOTHER EXERCISE SYSTEM FROM THE FAR EAST

T'ai chi is the gracefully flowing exercise form that you may have seen being done by Chinese people in news or documentary footage. In China, people often gather in the morning, sometimes in a park or often at work, to do t'ai chi together.

T'ai chi is only one of a myriad of movement systems that the Chinese collectively refer to as Qigong, which means "working with energy." The now familiar martial arts of kung fu and karate are branches of this body of wisdom, and t'ai chi itself was originally considered a martial art. T'ai chi is now used more as a way of enhancing health and as a form of standing meditation. As a meditation, it helps to develop the mind by teaching the implicit unity of apparent opposites (yin and yang). It also teaches us that we are creatures between Heaven and Earth, with our feet firmly on the ground while we engage in fluid interaction with the air and sky. It allows us to express our personal power and to use it to create our own unique existences.

As a tool for well-being, t'ai chi has great potential as a system you can do at home. Though you would undoubtedly receive more benefit from taking a class, it's also possible to learn from a video. Since anyone can receive videos through the mail, there are no excuses about its availability.

T'ai chi is a non-impact activity. There is very little danger of hurting yourself (less than with self-taught yoga). Yet it provides many of the same benefits of yoga in terms of reducing stress.

Despite its exotic origins, t'ai chi is imminently practical. It doesn't take up a lot of space. It isn't noisy. In fact, it's perfectly quiet. That means you could do it any time of day or night without disturbing anyone else (for example, in hotel rooms while traveling). As with walking, the equipment (loose clothing and soft shoes) is minimal. It requires no memberships. T'ai chi has no stunningly beautiful people selling it via infomercials.

Because you do t'ai chi standing, you could practice it outside on your porch, in the backyard, or even at a park. But since most of us tend to be self-conscious about new exercise programs, it's reassuring to know it can be done in your bedroom, living room or den.

T'ai chi is said to lower blood pressure, reduce heart rate, and generally improve circulation (thereby increasing oxygen to the tissues). It is also said to enhance immunity and improve mood. Oriental medicine is an approach to healing which includes the belief that illness results when energy flow is blocked, causing imbalance. T'ai chi helps to keep this energy flowing.

Besides practicality, why might you choose t'ai chi? One reason could be that since you do this form of exercise standing, it is a weight-bearing exercise, which can help you avoid osteoporosis. It's simultaneously a low-impact form of exercise, meaning it won't be hard on your joints. The fact that it stimulates circulation in so many ways means it can also help prevent as well as minimize arthritis. Exercise is at the top of the list of how to reverse arthritis or minimize its symptoms.

WHERE TO STUDY T'AI CHI

To find a t'ai chi class, look in Adult Education catalogs, inquire at the YMCA, and check under "Martial Arts Instruction" in the Yellow Pages for a school. Your local library may have books and videos, and I found three different t'ai chi videos at my neighborhood video store. The Resources section offers suggestions for books, videos and a website on t'ai chi.

"Bodywork recharges oneself from a feeling of lethargy. And certainly, bodywork is about pleasure. "

Chapter Twenty-Seven

BODYWORK FEELS SOOO GOOD!

Use of massage to promote health and healing is so universal that it's impossible to say where and when it began. Cave paintings in the Pyrenees, dating back to 15,000 B.C., show that people were then using touch therapeutically. Did it exist prior to that? Undoubtedly, as it is an instinctual human response to rub a spot that hurts—with your own hand if you can reach it, or by asking someone else to help if you can't.

Ancient healers understood the value of massage. Hippocrates, called the Father of Western Medicine, wrote in the 4th century B.C. that "The physician must be acquainted with many things and assuredly with rubbing." Rome's Galen (131-200 A.D.), whose anatomical studies on animals and observations of how the human body functions dominated medical theory and practice in Europe until the Renaissance, discussed an early version of massage in his book, *De Sanitate Tuenda*.

What's new about massage is the respect it is now regaining as its effectiveness is validated by modern research techniques. Simultaneously its cost remains low relative to high-tech medical technologies. This, of course, causes insurance companies to sit up and take notice. They are becoming gradually more open to reimbursing its cost. When you have a physical complaint, ask your physician if massage therapy might be beneficial and if he or she would be willing to prescribe it. The answer may just be "yes." Massage is sometimes the most powerful therapeutic tool possible.

In the past century, as with so many other aspects of our lives, there has been an explosion of knowledge regarding massage (which is now referred to more broadly as bodywork). Different forms are used to achieve specific therapeutic goals. Problems that can be addressed with massage include pain, sports injuries and joint stiffness due to all forms of arthritis. Bodywork can also be used to help resolve emotional issues. In short, bodywork has become the most widely recognized and accepted form of alternative medicine. In general, the only downside to bodywork is that it can cause something that's happening in one part of the body to spread to another part. So if you have a serious chronic illness or inflammation, check with your physician.

Bodywork doesn't have to be about fixing a body that needs repair, however. It can be about maintaining and maximizing health, reducing the effects of stress, recharging oneself from a feeling of lethargy, expanding mind and spirit, or simply allowing oneself to be more present in the moment.

Bodywork is certainly about pleasure. I think most of us with hedonistic tendencies recognize that. I have come across the scientific explanation. It seems that therapeutic massage causes the release of endorphins and enkephalins, the body's natural opiates. For this reason, massage can become habit-forming.

This seems to be the epitome of luxurious relaxation. We see massage depicted in popular culture as something that powerful business people, crime figures, entertainment execs and athletes do routinely, even at the office, where they always seem to receive an important call while on the massage table. If I were rich and powerful, I would say to my assistant, "Tell Mr. Eisner I'll call him back tomorrow." But I am not among the aforementioned. Other than a couple of greatly appreciated gift-certificate massages, the majority of my personal experiences with massage came as part of my treatments for whiplash after being rear-ended three times in five years. (That's life in Los Angeles as I have experienced it.) The chiropractors managed to straighten out my neck, but the massage felt like a true consolation prize. Massage does console, so if you ever need a gift idea for a friend who's going through a difficult time, a gift certificate for a massage could be very thoughtful. (The "friend" could even be you.)

SWEDISH MASSAGE

Swedish massage has a fascinating history. Its principles as a Western healing modality were established by Per Heinrik Ling, a Swedish clergyman's son who traveled all over Europe seeking a cure for his rheumatoid arthritis. It is unclear whether he actually went to China, or based his system on a translation of an ancient Chinese text called *The Cong-Fou of the Tao-Tse* that he found in France. Nonetheless, Ling used his newfound knowledge of the Chinese techniques to overcome his arthritis. Returning to Sweden, Ling incorporated the ancient knowledge with information on circulation discovered by William Harvey about 150 years before. In 1816, Ling established The Royal Institute of Gymnastics in Stockholm where his "Swedish movement treatment" was employed for healing. Though not initially accepted by the medical establishment, over the years, documentation of its effectiveness was accumulated. By the end of Ling's life, it had been widely recognized. This was an early milestone in the integration of "modern" science and ancient healing arts that we now call complementary medicine.

Those popular depictions of massage, with the kneading of the back muscles, the oil, the towels—that's Swedish massage. It is the form most often done in spas and health clubs for purposes of stress reduction and relaxation.

Swedish massage is the massage form from which the majority of new techniques have sprung. However, because most of these new techniques are used therapeutically, they are beyond the scope of this book. In his book, *BodyWork: What Type of Massage to Get—and How to Make the Most of It*, Thomas Claire discusses a great number of them. His book is now considered a reference book that clarifies many of the subtle differences between one style of bodywork and another. You may be able to find a copy of Claire's book at your local library.

Among these many massage modalities, there is one I want to make sure you're aware of. It's reflexology. Why? Well, reflexology has the unusual characteristic of being something you can do on your own body. It's certainly something you can learn to do with and for your family and/or mate.

REFLEXOLOGY

Reflexology is a form of massage that concentrates on the feet, though it can be done on the hands and ears as well. It's based on the concept that the essential parts of the body, such as limbs and organs, are associated with specific areas of the feet, hands, ears and skin. These are called reflex spots, hence the name, *"reflexology."* When a spot on the foot, hand or ear is massaged, it prompts a change in the corresponding organ, gland or limb. Reflexology is the therapeutic art and science of deliberately effecting positive physical change by knowing where and how to massage the feet, hands, etc. This is not a new therapy. Ancient Chinese and Egyptian "foot maps" have been found.

Reflexology uses a zone system similar to that on which acupuncture and acupressure are based. It divides the body into 10 different zones, five on each side of the midpoint of the body. The same zones divide the feet and hands. If an organ or nerve is in Zone 3 of the body, it will be in Zone 3 of the feet and hands. Reflexology improves energy flow by loosening blockages in the feet. In doing so, it will increase energy flow to other organs and limbs in the same zone.

Thomas Claire reports in his *Bodywork* book cited above that "a quarter of the bones in our body are in our feet—26 bones, 33 joints, 19 muscles, 107 ligaments and *more than 7,000 nerve endings* in each foot." Feet are more sensitive in cultures where they are kept covered.

We've become divorced from our feet. Not so with children, who love to go barefoot and often can't be stopped from abandoning footwear. Children are still in touch with the fact that our feet are our connection to Earth. To understand how such a relatively simple activity as massaging the feet can have a tremendously powerful effect on health, we need to increase our appreciation of the role our feet play. Among mammals, one of our most distinguishing features is our upright posture and our ability to achieve locomotion using only two feet rather than four. This frees up our hands and makes it possible for us to use our opposable thumb and forefinger. (And this is why, as we say in our house, "primates rule, dogs drool.")

You probably haven't thought much about the role of

TIPS FOR SELECTING A MASSAGE THERAPIST

When choosing a massage therapist, here are a few points to remember:

- If you have a preference regarding the sex of the massage therapist, be certain to mention it.
- You can find a well-qualified massage therapist by asking for a referral from a holistically-oriented health practitioner.
- If you don't know any holistic health practitioners, look up chiropractors in the Yellow Pages. They often work with massage therapists.
- Check the Yellow Pages to see if there's a massage school in the area. If so, you may be able to enjoy quality massage at a bargain price if you're willing to be someone the students train on.
- Be wary of ads for massage. It could be a "massage parlor" (i.e., sexual massage).
- If you want massage principally for relaxation and well-being, a health club can set up an appointment, especially if you're a member.
- A good day spa will have a competent massage therapist.
- If friends have ever mentioned having a massage, ask who they recommend.

You have every right to inquire regarding the training, experience and professional affiliations of a massseur/masseuse. The website of the American Massage Therapy Association can provide references for well-trained therapists. (See Resources.)

your feet in all this evolutionary progress. Well, the feet function as a sensory organ, gathering information so rapidly and quietly that we rarely think about it—unless we step on something disruptive. Any variation in our working surface is communicated instantly through our feet to the brain. For the most part, we unconsciously adjust our stride and our balance to compensate for the surface on which we're walking. Think of how we step off curbs, walk down stairs, go around mud puddles and cross ice. Unless something causes pain to the foot, we hardly notice all the changes our feet encounter. Yet each of those different surfaces requires responses from our brain that are sent to the muscles via the central nervous system, and to the organs via the autonomic nervous system.

Our feet encounter a lot of stress because they carry the weight of the body, concentrated by the force of gravity, onto the relatively small surface area of our feet. This pressure is compounded by unyielding surfaces such as concrete, stone and tile. Even many interior surfaces in the workplace or in our kitchens are hard. Just to massage the feet in general relieves pressure and promotes circulation.

A couple of warnings: If you're diabetic, you should not do reflexology on the feet. The reason? Well, diabetes often causes damage to the capillaries and nerves of the feet. A diabetic could, however, benefit from hand reflexology. (See Resources.) If you're pregnant, remember the feet contain nerve endings for all the organs in your body. Too much pressure on the nerves related to the reproductive system could conceivably cause miscarriage, so caution is advised —better to rely on the services of a professional reflexologist rather than experiment on yourself.

I can only touch on the subject of reflexology here, but

for those interested in more information, there are wonderful books available. (See Resources.) If you just want to achieve a bit of stimulation to your feet, you can use various tools, sandals, bathmats and foot-bathing systems that provide a gentle approximation of reflexology. The cheapest and most enjoyable is a barefoot walk on a sandy beach. These approaches are not as specific as true reflexology, but that doesn't matter if your goal is just to achieve a nonspecific enhancement of health and pleasure. Most of these approaches are inexpensive. Treat yourself and enjoy!

If you're interested in a greater or more specific effect, I recommend you buy a reflexology book and a chart of the feet. Then proceed gently and cautiously. If you find areas of your feet that are extremely sensitive, do not continue to apply pressure to them. You would do well, however, to report the sensitivity to a *licensed* holistically-oriented healthcare professional to help you identify the reason for the sensitivity, as it could indicate a serious problem. Note: A reflexologist cannot legally diagnose in any way.

Hand reflexology is a fascinating subject. Learning how to administer reflexology to your hands presents a fabulous opportunity to find something truly useful to do while on "hold," or during long meetings and conference calls. Think of being able to discreetly give yourself a massage during such tedious occasions. If you don't already use a headset, this could be the excuse you're looking for to invest in one, along with a book on hand reflexology.

A professional reflexologist can show you how to massage your own feet or hands, and your mate's. This bit of training could be well worth the cost of paying for a professional's time. Weekend workshops to learn reflexology are available, but you might need to be in a major met-

NEW TO MASSAGE?

If you've never experienced a professional massage, here are some tips that will help keep the experience a good one.

- Carve out time for the massage. Don't make the appointment too close to a meal, either before or after, and certainly try to avoid having to rush off to another engagement right away. You'll want to either ease back into your schedule, or plan the time to go home and relax or nap.

- You'll be asked to remove your clothing other than your underwear. If you're uncomfortable with this, just say so. Also remove jewelry and contact lenses.

- The masseur/masseuse will probably keep your body draped, other than the part being worked on. If not and you become cold, just say so.

- Talk about your preferences. If you prefer non-fragrant oil, mention it. If you don't wish to talk during the session, the massage therapist won't be offended. If something feels uncomfortable, speak up. In general, feel free to voice your concerns. The therapist wants your experience to be positive.

ropolitan area to find one. Taking such a workshop, however, would certainly provide you with sufficient training to work successfully on yourself, your mate and/or family.

Reflexology does not involve disrobing and this characteristic improves its accessibility. People who have not experienced bodywork in the past may be reluctant to climb onto a massage table practically naked and have someone they don't know work on their muscles. With reflexology, you need only take off your socks and shoes. This does not diminish the effect. Even experienced bodyworkers can be surprised at reflexology's effectiveness. Laura Norman, one of the country's leading reflexologists, and a student of Swedish massage, shiatsu and many other bodywork modalities, has commented "...in my experience, nothing can induce such a deep state of relaxation as reflexology."

ADDED PLEASURES

All forms of bodywork combine beautifully with aromatherapy. It's an easy thing to do, as you only need to add a few drops of essential oil to a massage oil to combine the two. In fact, now that you understand their therapeutic benefits, just think of how much enjoyment you can get from combining massage and aromatherapy with music and soft lighting. What a gift for yourself and those you love!

*"Saunas are profoundly beneficial. If you can find a place
nearby and develop the habit of taking a regular sauna,
it will have a tremendous effect on your health."*

Chapter Twenty-Eight

SPA CULTURE WITHOUT BIG BUCKS

Going to a spa is a trendy thing for affluent folks to do
these days. Alas, I'm not among them. But I have good news
regarding spa culture! It's something you can enjoy, on a
regular basis, without *beaucoup* bucks.

There are three topics in this chapter. The first part is
about saunas. The second is on how to create a spa experience at home. The last section looks at finding affordable
spas. (They do exist!)

SAUNA SECRETS

I'm initially emphasizing saunas because they're profoundly beneficial. If you can find a place nearby and develop the habit of taking a regular sauna, it will have a tremendous effect on your health—both on a mental and physical level.

When I refer to a sauna, I mean a dry-heat room, with
wood benches, kept at a temperature of about 165°. At that
temperature, the body quickly begins to sweat.

Saunas are one of the most enjoyable ways I've discovered to detox. The skin is the body's largest organ and primary routes for detoxification. During a sauna, toxins come
out through the skin as an element of perspiration.

The Finns have been doing saunas for a long time. I once experienced a Finnish style sauna in a posh little ski "shack." Adjacent to the sauna was an uncovered porch where the snow accumulated. Between periods in the sauna, we would throw ourselves into the snow, just like the Finns. The Finns are also known to jump into an icy lake to end the sauna! This is an experience worthy of all true thrill-seekers.

Native American sweat lodges are similar to saunas, but they're used for spiritual as well as physical purification. Techniques for inducing perspiration are also part of the Ayurvedic tradition of medicine in India. We're only now beginning to fully appreciate these ancient techniques.

Gaining access to a sauna was what caused me to join a gym a couple of years ago. It must have been 30 years since I'd belonged to one. You have probably noticed that gyms have special offers all the time. You can shop for a good deal, but it's important to choose a gym you like. Find one that is convenient and well-maintained, otherwise you won't want to go. Mine is far from luxurious, but the friendliness of the staff makes up for that. Plus, it's a bargain—I pay only $19 a month. I figure if I go just once a week and do nothing more than take a sauna, it's well worth it.

Many hotels now have saunas, and you may be able to arrange to use theirs as a non-guest. This is also true about their swimming pools. I suggest you call the hotel manager's office and be ready to negotiate. Hotels are often interested in finding additional income to offset their many expenses, but it may not be a request they receive every day.

It's also possible to buy a sauna unit for your home. I've listed a couple of manufacturers in Resources. I'm not saying this is an inexpensive route to take. However, if you use it several times a week, or if more than one person in the household takes saunas on a regular basis, it would certainly be worth the money.

If you fellow workaholics need further justification for spending the time, I might mention that it's easy to read in a dry sauna, so there's some multi-tasking that can be accomplished. In fact, I think it's a great place to read, because it detracts me from thinking about how warm I'm feeling. I've experimented with several types of reading material. I recommend racy biographies if you're not trying to keep up with your reading of newspapers and trade magazines.

Saunas are not recommended for some types of people. These categories include pregnant women, or women who might be pregnant. There is some disagreement about whether it might be harmful in early pregnancy, but if you're in that category, why take a chance? Saunas are not universally recommended for persons with high blood pressure or heart disease. Still, some books say saunas are helpful because they allow blood vessels to expand, thereby improving circulation. I urge you to consult your physician if you're in that category.

If you're very toxic from known chemical exposure, this can be an effective way to help regain your health—however, you must be under supervision. I've included a list of sauna therapists in Resources.

Saunas require you to use your own good judgment. Over a period of time, you can build up to rather long periods in the sauna, with great results. But you need to do that gradually. When you first begin doing saunas, stay in until you begin to feel uncomfortable. Initially, this might only be 5 or 10 minutes. If you find yourself becoming lightheaded or nauseous, it's definitely time to quit for the day.

After your sauna, take a shower. End the shower with cold water, even if it's only for a couple of seconds. Sometimes, I go back into the sauna. I always finish with a hot shower, followed by a brief cold shower.

Always drink a lot of water before and during your sauna, with a strong recommendation that it's filtered or distilled water. I can easily drink more than a quart of water in a half hour in the sauna. Taking a good vitamin and mineral supplement is also a good idea. It helps the detoxification process that's being stimulated and makes sure that you're not losing too much potassium via perspiration. Eating a banana before you go in can also help keep your potassium level high.

As part of the shower, wash your hair to remove toxins from your scalp. Use clean towels and then throw them in the dirty clothes hamper—they're now holding some toxins that have come out of your body.

Another terrific benefit of a long sauna is coming out of it marvelously relaxed. It's that same warm jellyfish feeling I experience from yoga.

You can further increase that feeling of relaxation by scheduling a *massage* after your sauna. It's a perfect time because the sauna has already done a lot of the work. Your whole body is warmed up. The blood is circulating well. You're already relaxed. The masseur/masseuse will then be able to take you to an even deeper level of benefit. The bodywork helps stimulate circulation in general and that of the lymph system in particular. It can help to break up deposits of toxins that may be contributing to joint stiffness. Your gym may be able to set up an appointment for you with a qualified masseur/masseuse. And even if you can only afford to do this occasionally, after the first time I won't have to tell you why you might want to do it as often as possible.

But back to the sauna and the hot and cold shower routine. Remember to always start with hot water and end with cold. Initially, you might resist the idea of using the cold water rinse. However, after a sauna your body is so warm, I promise you that the cold water won't make you feel uncomfortable. Instead you'll feel breathlessly exhilarated.

According to Drs. Bennett and Barrie, authors of the *7-Day Detox Miracle*, there's a marvelous sequence of events that makes the sauna and shower totally worthwhile. The heat stimulates the immune system and causes white blood cells to travel into the tissues where they clean up toxins, metabolic waste, bacteria and even viruses. Heat also relaxes and soothes the body.

Then the cold invigorates the body and can reduce inflammation, which is the body's reaction to injury, manifested by pain, heat, swelling and redness. The alternation between hot and cold will stimulate the adrenal glands and the endocrine system. It can reduce congestion and activate organ function. It's excellent for stimulating circulation to the digestive system and the liver. This, in turn, is helpful to detoxification, which happens on several levels during this sauna and hot/cold shower process.

All in all, it's very cleansing for the body. And you will be able to feel it immediately. This is definitely on the list of my highest recommendations for both pleasure and benefit. Frankly, once you find a place to take a sauna, and somehow manage to make the time to go there, it's a rather passive activity. You don't have to exercise before the sauna. You might feel like a little walk after the sauna because you'll be so relaxed and the breeze will feel so good. If it's cold outside, make sure you're bundled up so you don't become chilled.

AT-HOME SPA TECHNIQUES

Women's magazines regularly include articles with at-home spa techniques, and maybe you've tried some of them.

Okay, men, maybe you haven't. But you could. Spas that cater to men are all the rage, so you could do this for yourself without any apologies.

In addition to what's already been mentioned in Chapter 16 on bathing, a few of my favorite techniques are mentioned below. These are not merely pleasurable, they are even beneficial to your health!

These are especially nice as a way to luxuriate at home on days when you don't feel like going out. They also make a great complement to the detox weekend strategy. Either component is excellent, but doing both should make you feel like you've been on vacation (or at a spa) for a week.

TURN YOUR BATHROOM INTO A STEAM ROOM

Yes, you can experience a steam room effect right at home. Here's how:

1. Fill a handkerchief with fragrant herbs, such as lavender, mint or eucalyptus. (See if you can find something aromatic in the garden. Otherwise, the health food store will have aromatic teas sold in bulk that can be used.) Tie the hankerchief and herbs into a ball and then tie that onto the showerhead fixture so that the shower spray will dampen it.
2. Close the bathroom door and windows, and even plug up the crack under the door.

3. Turn on the shower as hot as possible for 10 minutes.
4. Turn off the water and sit in the steam for another 10 minutes. This is a good time for a hair treatment or facial.
5. Take a warm shower and rub your skin vigorously with a sisal mitt.
6. Finish with a quick cold shower.

AROMATHERAPY SALT MASSAGE

Note: Some readers may prefer to take a quick shower before doing the salt massage.

Stir a quarter cup of water into two cups of coarse sea salt, then add a few drops of your favorite essential oil. I love lavender. Clove oil is another favorite. Wonderful essential oil blends can also be purchased. Fill the bathtub with a few inches of warm water. Step in, and after splashing water up onto your legs, begin with your ankles and rub the salt vigorously all over your legs. Next, do the same with your arms. Then wet your chest, back, buttocks and abdomen and rub salt over all the spots you can reach. Then fill the tub with safely hot water and relax for a few minutes. The salt is detoxifying. Then rinse your body first with warm water and then with cool water.

In addition to stimulating circulation and exfoliating, the surprising benefit of a salt rub is that it softens your skin. This is one of those techniques that's nice to do before you go to bed. It may cause you to perspire quite a bit, so you will probably want to keep a glass of water by your bed. In the morning, take a shower and apply moisturizer.

FACIAL SAUNA

There's nothing new about this technique, but it's wonderful for your skin. It's also something you can easily do at the kitchen table on a weeknight after the supper dishes have been put away. Bring a large pot of water to a boil, and throw in a couple of peppermint or spearmint teabags or add a couple of drops of a favorite essential oil to the water. A calming blend would be good. Place the pot with a cover on a hotpad or potholder on the table. Wrap your hair in a towel. Now remove the cover. With a second towel, form a tent over the water and just breathe in the steam for five minutes or longer. Talk about small luxuries being beneficial! This takes so little time and can have great benefit. This easy facial sauna will relax you all over. It will also improve your skin and help to clear your sinuses.

FACIAL MASQUES

You can use any number of commercial facial masques after a sauna. But here are some great, easy homemade masques. Remember to be careful around your eyes; facial masques should not be used above the upper part of your cheekbones or below the brows. (See "Two Simple Eye Treatments" on next page.) A good time to lie back and relax is while you're letting the facial masque dry.

Try this facial if you have *dry skin*. Mix equal parts of avocado and mayonnaise into a paste. Apply to your face, and rest for a half hour while also doing the cucumber or tea-bag eye treatment. Rinse your face, use toner and moisturize.

For *oily skin*, here's a different masque. Whip together two egg whites and a teaspoon each of lemon juice and vinegar. Then brush it onto your face. Now rest for a half hour

TWO SIMPLE EYE TREATMENTS

You can give your eyes a nice simple treatment in one of two ways. One is to place fresh *cucumber slices*, about a quarter inch thick, over your eyes. They're very cooling. Leave them on your eyes until the facial masque is dry.

The second option is to use *tea bags*. They don't have to be any special kind, just orange pekoe or black tea is fine. First, wet them. Then, put them in the freezer for a half hour or so. Remove and let them thaw slightly so there's no worry of freezer burn. Finally, lie down and place the bags over your closed eyelids. The tea bags feel marvelous, soften your skin, and reduce puffiness. They also help minimize dark circles. The cost/benefit ratio is pretty high on this one.

while also enjoying an eye treatment. Rinse your face, use toner and moisturize.

In terms of ease of preparation and cost-effectiveness of ingredients, my favorite home facial masque is a paste of *oatmeal and water*. Stir them together until the mixture is nice and gooey. I like the contrast here. You go from the absolutely splendid form of simple relaxation with the facial sauna to applying gooey oatmeal paste to your face. Warning: You're sure to look funny with the oatmeal drying. It feels like you've become the villain in a horror movie. Your kids will think this is the funniest thing they've ever seen. (If laughing with them about this kind of stuff isn't your idea of fun, you might want to do this after they've gone to bed or when they're not at home.) But after it's dried and you've scraped it off and washed your face, you'll be amazed at how soft and radiant your skin is.

Each one of these facials is wonderful to do before going out for a special occasion. You can also do them in the evening as a way to relax while listening to great music.

Other sources of information for spa-at-home ideas are listed in Resources.

OTHER AFFORDABLE SPA EXPERIENCES

The *"day spa"* idea is the rage in the beauty services business. A day spa, is differentiated from a destination spa, which falls under the category of "resort" in the Yellow Pages. Day spas represent a great expansion of consciousness as to what beauty is and how beneficial it can be to incorporate many of the health-promoting techniques discussed in this book, including massage, aromatherapy and hydrotherapy.

Finding a favorite day spa may take a bit of effort. As you check them out, you'll find all sorts of facilities. Some will be lovely, others will be disappointing. There will be all sorts of personnel, services and promises. The beauty treatments can definitely make you feel pampered. To discuss whether the various skin treatments that day spas offer can make you look younger would require another book. If you're skeptical, you're less likely to be disappointed. Ask about the experience and credentials of the *"aesthetician"* (the person who performs skin enhancement treatments) and the masseur/masseuse. Compare prices. If you find a place you like with reasonable prices, that's great. If you don't, there are additional spa experiences to seek out.

I also encourage you to search your geographical vicinity for *old spas* (destination spas) and *hot springs*. In numerous areas of the country, there are spas that have been around for 50 to 100 years at natural hot springs. If there's a place called Hot Springs in your state, check it out. There may be an old spa there. You can also check it out via the Internet by searching on "hot springs" + "[your state]" + "spa." Also, ask the Auto Club or your travel agent.

Here are some of the bargain-shopper destination spas in my home state of California:

- Glen Ivy, near Corona, California, is $35/day weekends and $25/day weekdays for access to hot springs, saunas, mud baths and swimming pools; other services are extra. This is a beautifully maintained "mature" facility. (See *www.glenivy.com*.)

- The Desert Hot Springs Spa Hotel, near Palm Springs, California, has day rates for their pools and dry sauna of only $5 to $7 a person. (This is not a typo. See *www.dhsspa.com*.)

- Calistoga Spa Hot Springs of Napa Valley in Northern California is not cheap, but not that expensive for a special occasion either. It's $50 a day for the mud baths and about $100 if you have a full massage. (See *www.calistogaspa.com*.)

Another approach would be to call massage therapists listed in your phone book, or in the state listings for the massage association, and ask them if they know of a nice affordable spa, preferably an old one. Admittedly, this isn't going to be as convenient as your local hairdresser's salon. However, the atmosphere of being outdoors in a real hot-spring-fed pool in a beautiful old facility is an authentic experience to which a day spa can never come close.

BE GOOD TO YOU

Whatever type of facility you use, including your home, the spa experience makes a good gift to yourself. If you combine it with knowledge of mild personal detox, it will not only be intensely pleasurable, but also extremely beneficial.

"It doesn't matter whether you implement a close approximation of the ideas in the book, or if they simply inspire you to figure out what works for you."

ON MOVING FORWARD

I'd like to share with you the feeling of being able to write the conclusion to my first book and then tell you, briefly, how it might relate directly to you.

I'm proud to have reached this point, and more than a little relieved. Writing a book takes more than just the time used in front of the computer to get the words down on paper. It absorbs all available time and energy from every other aspect of your life. Writing a book cannot be accomplished without sacrificing time that would have been devoted to other income-producing activities, hobbies or obligations. It certainly redirects time normally spent with friends and family. The process has taken longer than I thought it would, but most things in life seem to go that way. The good news is that this project is turning out better than I thought it would, and creating the book has been an amazing experience.

Over the past year, I went from having an idea to seeing it become what it is now. As I write this, the project is very close to realization. The words have been composed. The cover has been designed and redesigned. A plan for launching the book is in the works.

In terms of being able to commit words to paper or an

electronic screen, I knew I was capable of writing a book. I've done a lot of writing for a long time. But when it came time to actually begin writing the book, to actually sit down and do it, I experienced a lot of anxiety. I didn't know how to begin. There were a number of false starts. If the truth be told, a lot of pages that I thought might be included in the book were later tossed.

The sections of the book that you now see as "Welcome to the Banquet" and Chapter One were not the first pages I wrote. Material that is now part of the middle of the book was the first to survive all the editing and tossing.

My advice to you, in terms of seeking greater health and balance, is to grab hold wherever you can, as I did in writing this book, and go from what you know. And if you experience a few false starts, don't be discouraged.

Another critical element was the words of a close friend who is a fine artist himself. As I anguished about how to begin this formidable task, he told me, artist to artist, to "trust the process." I didn't quite know what that meant, but he was so confident about this that some of it rubbed off.

Those three words, "trust the process," are the second part of what I want to pass along to you. For any of us to do something new requires an element of faith.

If you're already engaged in aspects of hedonistic self-care, it will probably be fairly easy for you to experiment with new techniques. But if you never have, practice the art of trust. You may have false starts. Some things might not work for you. Keep experimenting.

It's my great hope that this book will stimulate you to find more fun, energy and balance in life. It doesn't matter whether you can implement a close approximation of the ideas in the book, or if they simply inspire you to figure out what works for you.

I don't think life is a picnic, but I certainly believe we should all count our many blessings and schedule as many picnics as possible. We must trust that our experiences are leading us in a positive direction, even when the day-to-day experience seems far from positive or certain aspects and events cause great emotional, physical or financial difficulty. Again, trust the process.

We are all evolving. Change is the only constant. Consciousness, even when suppressed, never goes backward. These are universal truths.

Persevere!

Part Five

More Help for You

Notes

This section provides additional information about quotations, books and studies mentioned in *The Healthy Hedonist*.

CHAPTER 2. *The Dry Well*
Codependent No More: How to Stop Controlling Others and Start Caring for Yourself, Melody Beattie, A Hazelden Book, Harper San Francisco, 1987, p. 32.

CHAPTER 3. *The Lost Key*
Rem B. Edwards, Ph.D., *Pleasures and Pains: A Theory of Qualitative Hedonism,* Cornell University Press, Ithaca, NY, 1979.

CHAPTER 4. *Pillars of Healthy Hedonism*
Harlow, H.F., Harlow, M.K., Suomi, S.J., "From thought to therapy: lessons from a primate laboratory," *American Scientist,* Sept-Oct. 1971; 59(5): 538-549.

Vaillant, George E., M.D., and Mukamal, Kenneth, M.D., "Successful Aging," *American Journal of Psychiatry,* June 2001; 158 (6): 839-847.

Larson, D.B., Koenig, H.G., "Is God good for your health? The role of spirituality in medical care," Cleveland Clinic Journal of Medicine, February 2000: 67 (2): 80, 83-84.

CHAPTER 7. *Walk, Walk, Walk—Around the Block*
Gerber, M., Boutron-Ruault, M.C., Hercberg, S.,

Riboili, E., Scalbert, A., Siess, M.H., "Food and cancer: state of the art about the protective effect of fruits and vegetables," *Bulletin of the American Society for the Control of Cancer*, March 2002; 89(3): 293-312.

In an analysis of the health habits of 70,000 nurses over the past 25 years, researchers from the Harvard School of Public Health found that just 30 minutes a day of brisk walking or the equivalent will cut the odds of heart trouble, diabetes and various cancers, as well as boost longevity. The results of the study, known as the "Harvard Nurses' Health Study," became the basis for the book, *Healthy Women, Healthy Lives*, published by Simon & Schuster.

In an article by Mack Fenton titled "Walk your Way to Extra Energy," JoAnn Manson, M.D., one of the researchers on the Harvard Nurses' Health study, said, "Many people assume that exercise needs to be vigorous and lengthy to be beneficial, but walking as little as 10 minutes a day has proved to be much better than doing nothing at all." The article appeared in *New Choices*, March 2002, pp. 30-33. Fenton, is the author of *The Complete Guide to Walking for Health, Weight Loss and Fitness* (Lyon's Press).

In a *Time* magazine cover story, "The Science of Staying Healthy," January 21, 2002, Dr. Manson said, "Regular physical activity is probably as close to a magic bullet as we will come in modern medicine... if everyone in the U.S. were to walk briskly 30 minutes a day, we could cut the incidence of many chronic diseases 30% to 40%."

Trejo, J.L., Carro, E., Torres-Aleman, I., "Circulating insulin-like growth factor I mediates exercise-induced increases in the number of new neurons in the adult hippocampus," *Journal of Neuroscience*, March 2001; 21(5): 1628-34.

CHAPTER 9. *Rediscovering Energy*

Baker, Sidney MacDonald, M.D., *The Circadian Prescription*, A Perigee Book, published by The Berkley Publishing Group, a division of Penguin Putnam Inc., New York, NY, 2000, pp. 30-32.

Anderson, J.W., Johnstone, B.M., Cook-Newell M.E., "Meta-Analysis of the Effects of Soy Protein Intake on Serum Lipids," *New England Journal of Medicine*, 333: 276-282, August 3, 1995.

Jacobsen, B.K., Knutsen, S.F., Fraser, G.E., "Does high soy milk intake reduce prostate cancer incidence? The Adventist Health Study," *Cancer Causes & Control*, December 1998; 9(6): 553-7.

Severson, R.K., Nomura, A.M., Grove, J.S., Stemmermann, G.N., "A prospective study of demographics, diet, and prostate cancer among men of Japanese ancestry in Hawaii," *Accomplishments in Cancer Research*, April 1, 1989; 49(7): 1857-60.

Albertazzi, P., Zanotti, L., Forini, E., De Aloysio, D., "The Effect of Dietary Soy Supplementation on Hot Flushes," *Journal of the American Medical Association*, 91 (1998): 6-11.

CHAPTER 14. *Mood-Altering Strategies*

"According to the survey, children whose families eat healthy together watched less television, were more likely to partake in arts and music after school, and excelled in arts and English." From a survey of family eating habits conducted by WestSoy, a division of The Hain Celestial Group, Uniondale, NY, as reported in *Whole Foods*, December 2001.

CHAPTER 15. *Gifts of the Magi, Gifts for You*
Holmes, C., Hopkins, V., Hensford, C., MacLaughlin, V., Wilkinson, D., Rosenvinge, H., "Lavender oil as a treatment for agitated behaviour in severe dementia: a placebo controlled study," *International Journal of Geriatric Psychiatry*, April 2002; 17(4): 305-8.

CHAPTER 16. *The New Art of Bathing*
7-Day Detox Miracle, Peter Bennett, N.D., Stephen Barrie, N.D., with Sara Faye, Prima Publishing, 1999, p. 78.
The Whole Way to Natural Detoxification, Jacqueline Krohn, M.D., Frances A. Taylor, M.A., Jinger Prosser, L.M.T., Hartley & Marks, 2000.

CHAPTER 18. *Sleep, Blissful Sleep*
Scheen, A.J., "Clinical study of the month. Does chronic sleep deprivation predispose to metabolic syndrome?" *Revue médicale de Liège*, November 1999; 54(11): 898-900.
Garfinkel, D., Zisapel, N., "The Use of Melatonin for Sleep," *Nutrition*, Vol. 14, January 1998, 53-55.

CHAPTER 25. *Detox Weekends*
Roan, Shari, "Detox Demystified," *Los Angeles Times*, Sept. 3, 2001.
Ling, Lisa, "Why I Spent a Week in the Desert Starving," *USA Weekend*, Sept. 7-9, 2001.
Geller, L.I., Gladkikh, L.N., and Griaznova, M.V., "Treatment of Fatty Hepatosis in Diabetics," *J Probl Endokrinol* (Russia), 39 (1993): 20-22.
Lang, I., Nekam, K., Deak, G., et al.,

"Immunomodulatory and Hepatoprotective Effects of In Vivo Treatment with Free Radical Scavengers," *Ital J Gastroenterol*, 22 (1990): 283-87.

Feher, J., Deak, G., Muzes, G., et. al., "Liver-Protective Action of Silymarin Therapy in Chronic Alcoholic Liver Diseases," *Orv Hetil* (Hungary), 130 (1989): 2723-27.

Salmi, H.A., Sarna, S., "Effect of Silymarin on Chemical, Functional, and Morphological Alterations of the Liver. A Double-blind Controlled Study," *Scand J Gastroenterol*, 17 (1982): 517-21.

Magliulo, E., Gagliardi, E B., and Fiori, G.P., "Results of a Double-blind Study on the Effect of Silymarin in the Treatment of Acute Viral Hepatitis, Carried Out at Two Medical Centres," *Med Klin* (Germany), 73 (1978): 1060-65.

Muzes, G., Deak, G., Lang, I., et al., "Effect of Silymarin (Legalon) Therapy on the Antioxidant Defense Mechanism and Lipid Peroxidation in Alcoholic Liver Disease (Double-blind Protocol)," *Orv Hetil* (Hungary), 131 (1990): 863-66.

Ferenci, P., Dragosics, B., Dittrich, H., Frank, H., et al., "Randomized Controlled Trial of Silymarin Treatment in Patients with Cirrhosis of the Liver," *J Hepatol* (Netherlands), 9 (1989): 105-13.

CHAPTER 27. *Bodywork Feels So Good!*

Eisenberg, D.M., Davis, R.B., Ettner, S.L., Appel, S., Wilkey, S., Van Rompay, M., Kessler, R.C. "Trends in alternative medicine use in the United States, 1990-1997," *JAMA* 280 (1993): 1569-75.

Resources

The following pages list purchasing information for products mentioned in *The Healthy Hedonist*, as well as books, websites and other sources that can provide additional information on the subjects covered in each of the chapters.

CHAPTER 2. *The Dry Well*
  Codependent No More: How to Stop Controlling Others and Start Caring for Yourself, Melody Beattie (Hazelden Information Education, 1996)
  Facing Codependence: What It Is, Where It Comes From, How It Sabotages Our Lives, Pia Mellody (Harper San Francisco, 1989)

CHAPTER 5. *Wake Me Gently, Please*
  Zen Clock by Now & Zen, $99.95, *www.now-zen.com* 800-779-6383
  Nature Sounds CD Player/Clock Radio by Timex, product #C76 691 4582T, $99.00, *Spiegel.com* 800-527-1577
  Sharper Image CD Radio/Alarm Clock with Sound Soother 20, product #S1687TNM, $219.95, *www.sharperimage.com* 800-344-4444
  Sky Mall, Bio-Brite's Sunrise Clock, product #88630A $99.95, *www.skymall.com*, 800-SKYMALL

CHAPTER 7. *Walk, Walk, Walk—Around the Block*
Resource for physiatrists (fizz ee at trists)
American Academy of Physical Medicine & Rehabilitation
www.aapmr.org/consumers/public/what.htm
Magnetic bike trainers, 800-NASHBAR
(800-627-4227)
Prayer Walk; Becoming a Woman of Prayer, Strength and Discipline, Janet McHenry (WaterBrook, 2001)
Peace Is Every Step, Thich Nhat Hanh (Bantam Books, 1992)
The Spirited Walker, Carolyn Kortge (Harper San Francisco, 1998)

CHAPTER 8. *Better Showering: Making the Most of a Good Thing*
Lymphatic Drainage Massage, a video produced by Real Bodywork (www.deeptissue.com) featuring Sean Riehl. This video (prepared to teach lymphatic drainage massage to massage therapists) includes an excellent introduction that explains the workings of the lymph system.

CHAPTER 9. *Rediscovering Energy*
Melissa Metcalfe, N.D.*
870-E Hampshire Rd., Westlake Village, CA 91361
dr.melissa@naturalsolutions.com, 805-374-7363
(*N.D. stands for naturopathic physician, a specialist in assessing and correcting biochemical imbalances using natural foods and supplements. Check the website for the American Association of Naturopathic Physicians, *www.aanp.org*, to find an N.D. near you.)

The Circadian Prescription, Sidney MacDonald Baker, M.D., with Karen Baar, M.P.H. (Perigee Book, 2000)

Amazing Soy, Dana Jacobi (Morrow, 2002)

The Whole Soy Cookbook, Patricia Greenberg (Three Rivers, 1998)

Soy Desserts, Patricia Greenberg (HarperCollins, 2002)

CHAPTER 11. *Work in Balance*

For soothing music, Peter Janson, *Sometimes From Here*, from Eastern Woods Music, *www.EasternWoodsMusic.com*

Don't Sweat the Small Stuff at Work: Simple Ways to Minimize Stress and Conflict While Bringing Out the Best in Yourself and Others, Richard Carlson (Hyperion, 1988)

Generations at Work: Managing the Clash of Veterans, Boomers, Xers, and Nexters in Your Workplace, Ron Zemke (AMACOM,1999)

How to Deal with Difficult People, a two-cassette audio seminar by Dr. Rick Brinkman and Dr. Rick Kirschner. From CareerTrack Audiotape Seminars, 3085 Center Green Drive, Boulder, CO 80301, 303-440-7440

A seminar on "Conflict Management Skills for Women" is presented for a reasonable cost on a regular basis in most U.S. metropolitan areas by Skillpath Seminars, *www.skillpath.com*, 800-873-7545.

CHAPTER 13. *Tasty, Right-Fat Snacks*

Microwave Chipmaker, from Ensar Corporation, Wheeling, IL 60090-6035

CHAPTER 14. *Mood-Altering Strategies*

Sounds of Healing, A Physician Reveals the Therapeutic Power of Sound, Voice, and Music, Mitchell L. Gaynor, M.D. (Broadway Books, 1999)

Sound Body, Sound Mind: Music for Healing by Andrew Weil, M.D. is designed to help draw a person into and through the entire range of brainwave states, from beta (the waking state,) down to alpha (the daydreaming and light meditation state), and then further down into theta (the level of the subconscious). Theta is generally only achieved in dreaming and deep meditation. Finally the listener goes down into delta, or deep sleep levels, with "just enough alpha to keep a link to the conscious mind," according to Dr. Weil's newsletter. The recording is available at bookstores and record stores, or directly from Upaya at 800-354-3943.

Steve Halpern, Ph.D., a pioneer in the therapeutic use of sound and music, has released more than 50 albums on his Inner Peace and SoundWave 2000 labels, designed to evoke a healing response in the listener. Visit *www.innerpeace.com*

The Ultimate Container Garden: All You Need to Know to Create Plantings for Spring, Summer, Autumn, and Winter, Stephanie Donaldson (Lorenz Books, 2001)

Outdoor Plants for Indoor Rooms, Kathy Sheldon (Lark Books, 2001)

Perfect Small Gardens, Peter McHoy (Lorenz Books, 2002)

Amaryllis bulbs are available October 23 through February 14 in a variety of pots, both plain and decorative, at prices ranging from $19.95 to $59.95 from Harry and David, *www.harryanddavid.com,* 800-547-3033.

Paper Whites in a blue delft-style bowl are available from September 15 through December for $16.99, from Figis, *www.figis.com*, 715-341-1363.

Four Months of Spring Color and Fragrance (December-March), $125, from Gardener's Supply Company, *www.gardeners.com*, 800-427-3363

CHAPTER 15. *Gifts of the Magi, Gifts for You*

A good resource for education in essential oil usage: Australasian College of Herbal Studies. *www.herbed.com*

A general commercial website for aromatherapy: *www.aromaweb.com*

A good source for oils: The Essential Oil Company *www.essentialoil.com,* 800-729-5912

Another good source for oils: Aura Cacia *www.auracacia.com*, 800-437-3301

The Complete Book of Essential Oils & Aromatherapy, Valerie Ann Worwood (New World Library, 1991)

The Essential Oils Book, Colleen K. Dodt (Storey Publishing, 1996)

Personalized Perfumes: More Than 40 Recipes for Making Fragrances with Essential Oils, Gail Duff (Simon & Schuster, 1994)

CHAPTER 16. *The New Art of Bathing*

The Healing Aromatherapy Bath, Margo Valentine Lazzara (Storey Publishing, 1999)

CHAPTER 17. *A Time of Peace*

The Art of Meditation, Joel S. Goldsmith (Harper & Row, 1956)

Meditation and Mantras, Swami Vishnu Devananda (OM Lotus Publishing Company, 1981)

The Relaxation Response, Herbert Benson, M.D. (William Morrow and Co., 1976)

20-Minute Retreats, Revive Your Spirits in Just Minutes a Day with Simple Self-Led Exercises, Rachael Harris, Ph.D. (Owl Books, 2000)

CHAPTER 18. *Sleep, Blissful Sleep*

No Time to Clean, How to Reduce & Prevent Cleaning the Professional Way, Don Aslett (Marsh Creek Press, 2000)

A Woman's Guide to Sleep, Guaranteed Solutions for a Good Night's Rest, Joyce A. Walsleben, Ph.D., and Rita Baron-Faust (Crown Publishers, 2000)

Learn to Sleep Well, A Practical Guide to Getting a Good Night's Rest, Chris Idzikowski. includes a 55-minute CD of visualizations, music and soothing ocean sounds. (Chronicle Books, 2000)

Mattress Buying Tips
www.mattress.com/service/6steps.asp
www.mattress.com/sleepwell/newmattress.asp

CHAPTER 19. *Good, Better, Best Weekends*

For more information on community supported agriculture (CSA):

Local Harvest, *www.localharvest.org*
Center for CSA Resources, *www.csacenter.org*
CSA resource list, *www.umass.edu/umext/csa*

CHAPTER 20. *Juicing & Saturday Salads*

The Juiceman's Power of Juicing, Jay Kordich (Warner Books, 1993)

Getting the Best Out of Your Juicer, William H. Lee, R.Ph., Ph.D. (Keats Publishing, 1992)

The Juicing Book, A Complete Guide to the Juicing of Fruits and Vegetables for Maximum Health and Vitality, Stephen Blaur (Avery, 1989)

CHAPTER 22. *Eating Out & Traveling*

Viva's Healthy Dining Guide, A Comprehensive Directory of Vegetarian, Healthy Ethnic, and Natural Foods Restaurants, and Markets Across America, Lisa Margolin and Connie Dee (Viva Center for Nutrition, Bridgewater, NJ, 2002)

Travel wardrobes from Travelsmith: *www.travelsmith.com*, 800-950-1600

CHAPTER 25. *Detox Weekends*

American Academy of Environmental Medicine is an association of physicians who treat people with health problems caused by adverse, allergic or toxic reactions to environmental substances. *www.aaem.com*, 316-684-5500

American Holistic Medical Association is an organization of licensed physicians who practice holistic medicine. *www.holisticmedicine.org*, 703-556-9245.

American Association of Naturopathic Physicians is an organization of licensed N.D.s who are graduates of certified North American universities offering four-year, postgraduate degrees in naturopathic medicine. *www.aanp.org*, 877-969-2267 toll-free.

American Osteopathic Association members, or D.O.s are fully licensed physicians, graduates of four-year medical schools who are able to prescribe medication and perform surgery. They treat holistically, using nontoxic and noninvasive therapies. *www.aoa-net.org*, 866-FIND-A-DO toll-free.

Jeffrey Bland, Ph.D., a renowned biochemist in the field of human nutrition, offers a free service to receive names of practitioners in your area who specialize in "functional medicine," a holistic medical approach that focuses on bodily function, including detoxification. 800-245-9076.

Detoxification & Healing: The Key to Optimal Health, Sidney MacDonald Baker, M.D. (Keats Publishing, Inc., 1997)

The 20-Day Rejuvenation Diet Program, Jeffrey Bland, Ph.D., with Sara Benum, M.A. (Keats Publishing, 1997)

7-Day Detox Miracle, Restore Your Mind and Body's Natural Vitality with This Safe and Effective Life-Enhancing Program, Peter Bennett, N.D., Stephen Barrie, N.D., Sara Faye, (Prima Health, a division of Prima Publishing, 1999)

Natural Detoxification, A Practical Encyclopedia, A Complete Guide to Clearing Your Body of Toxins, Jacqueline Krohn, M.D., Frances Taylor, M.A. (Hartley & Marks Publishers Inc., 2000)

The Detox Solution, The Missing Link to Radiant Health, Abundant Energy, Ideal Weight, and Peace of Mind, Patricia Fitzgerald (Illumination Press, 2001). *www.thedetoxsolution.com*

CHAPTER 26. *Yoga and T'ai Chi*
MAJOR YOGA DISCIPLINES

Sivananda Vedanta is one of several major international yoga organizations that teaches traditional yoga, emphasizing hatha yoga (the poses commonly associated with yoga) as a preparation for meditation and spiritual development. Beginners' classes are very gentle. Sivananda Vedanta's North American schools are located in Los Angeles, San Francisco, Grass Valley, CA, New York City, Woodbourne, NY, and Val-Morin, Quebec, Canada. *www.sivananda.org*, 800-469-9642.

Satchidananda Ashram is a second major international yoga organization, also emphasizing hatha yoga as a preparation for meditation and spiritual development. *www.yogaville.org*, 804-964-3221.

Iyengar Yoga was developed by B.K.S. Iyengar who, at 80, continues to teach in Pune, India. The tradition emphasizes precise alignment, facilitated with props such as straps, blocks and blankets. For the Iyengar Yoga Institute in San Francisco, *www.iyisf.org*

Ashtanga Yoga uses a vigorous, fast-paced series of sequential postures, of increasing difficulty, that allow students to work at their own pace. Students work up a sweat. *www.yogaworkshop.com*

Kundahlini Yoga is a vigorous system of yoga founded by Yogi Bhajan that incorporates postures, dynamic breathing techniques, chanting and meditation with the goal of awakening the individual's reservoir of cosmic energy. *www.3HO.org*

WEBSITES TO FIND A YOGA SCHOOL:
www.yogafinder.com
www.yogasite.com
www.yogajournal.com

BOOKS ON YOGA

Yoga: The Path to Holistic Health, B.K.S. Iyengar (DK Publishing, 2001)

Bikram's Beginning Yoga Class, Bikram Choudhury (J.P. Tarcher, 2000)

Yoga for Wimps, Poses for the Flexibly Impaired, Miriam Austin (Sterling Publications, 2000)

FOR YOGA VIDEOS AND DVDS

Visit *www.yogajournal.com* and click on the "Shop YJ" button to review a wide selection of videos and DVDs.

BOOKS ON T'AI CHI

The Healing Promise of Qi, Creating Extraordinary Wellness Through Qigong and Tai Chi, Roger Jahnke, O.M.D. (McGraw Hill, 2002)

The Compete Idiot's Guide to T'ai Chi & Qigong, Bill Douglas (2nd Edition, Alpha Books, 2002)

T'AI CHI VIDEOS

T'ai Chi for Health, Healing Arts, 800-722-7347

Discover Tai Chi, a series of videos by Natural Journeys. *www.naturaljourneys.com*, 800-737-1825

FOR MORE INFORMATION ON T'AI CHI & QIGONG:

National Qigong Association USA. *www.nqa.org*

CHAPTER 27. *Bodywork Feels Sooo Good!*

The New Sensual Massage: Learn to Give Pleasure With Your Hands, Gordon Inkeles (Arcata Arts, 1998)

Massage: The Ultimate Illustrated Guide, Clare Maxwell-Hudson, Sandra Lousada (DK Publishing, 1999)

Super Massage, Simple Techniques for Instant Relaxation, Gordon Inkeles and Sigga Bjornsson (Arcata Arts, 2001)

Hand Reflexology: Key to Perfect Health, Revised Edition, Mildred Carter, Tammy Weber, Z. Hussain (Prentice Hall Press, 2000)

Hand and Foot Reflexology: A Self-Help Guide, Kevin Kunz (Simon & Schuster, 1992)

The Busy Person's Guide to Reflexology, Simple Treatments and Five-Minute Routines, Ann Gillanders (Barrons Educational Series, 2002)

TO FIND A REFLEXOLOGIST:

The International Institute of Reflexology
www.reflexology-usa.net, 813-343-4811

TO FIND A MASSAGE THERAPIST:

American Massage Therapy Association
www.amtamassage.org, 708-864-0123

Associated Bodywork & Massage Professionals
www.abmp.com, 800-458-2267, 303-674-8478

CHAPTER 28. *Spa Culture without Big Bucks*
MANUFACTURERS

Health Mate Saunas. 800-946-6001

Air Wall Sauna. *www.awsauna.com,* 888-972-8627

Steam Embrace, *www.steamembrace.com,* 800-231-7832

Heavenly Heat Saunas, *www.pulseparty.com*
800-5SAUNAS,
Aroma Spa, *www.aromaspa.com*, 800-800-7222

DETOXIFICATION CLINICS

Center for Environmental Medicine
  North Charleston, SC, 843-572-1600
Environmental Health Center, Dallas, TX
  214-368-4132
Healing Naturally, Kirkland, WA, 425-821-8118
Preventive Medical Center of Marin, San Rafael, CA
  415-472-2343
Robbins Environmental Medicine Clinic
  Boca Raton, FL , 561-395-3282
Los Alamos Medical Center, Los Alamos NM
  505-662-9620

SPA-AT-HOME IDEA BOOKS

The Herbal Home Spa, Greta Breedlove (Storey Books, 1998)

Making Aromatherapy Creams & Lotions, Donna Maria (Storey Books, 2000)

Anti-Wrinkle Treatments for Perfect Skin, Pierre Jean Cousin (Storey Books, 2001)

HOT SPRINGS AND TRADITIONAL SPAS BOOKS

Touring California and Nevada Hot Springs, Matt Bischoff (FalconGuide, 1997)

Touring Montana and Wyoming Hot Springs, Jeff Birkby (FalconGuide, 1997)

Hot Springs & Hot Pools of the Northwest: Jayson Loam's Original Guide, Marjorie Gersh-Young (Aqua Thermal Access, 1999)

Beautiful Spas and Hot Springs of California, Melba Levick, photographer, and Stanley Young, text (Chronicle Books, 1998)

Recipes

I would like to share some of my favorite recipes with you, in hopes you'll share some of your favorites on The Healthy Hedonist, website *www.healthyhedonist.com.*

Let's start with two important recipes I make often. I hope you'll find them very useful.

TWO YOU'LL USE AGAIN & AGAIN

JB'S ENERGY BARS

1/4 cup of shredded coconut
3 tablespoons of organic sugar
3/4 cup of instant organic oatmeal
2 cups of pure water
1 cup of prunes or other dried fruit
grated rind of one orange
2 tablespoons of cocoa
1 1/4 cup of unsweetened applesauce
3/4 cup tahini
1/4 cup maple syrup (optional)
3 cups soy protein powder
Plus topping ingredients (see next page)

Spray two 8" square baking pans with an all-natural non-stick cooking spray (available from a health food store). Dust the pans with organic sugar, then with a thin layer of un-sweetened coconut.

In a double-boiler, combine the oatmeal and water and

cook over medium heat for about 10 minutes. Meanwhile, chop the prunes in a mini-food processor, adding a sprinkle of protein powder to help keep the prunes from becoming so sticky they won't chop.

Add the prunes, tahini, applesauce, maple syrup, cocoa and orange rind to the oatmeal mixture. Stir until well mixed.

Add the protein powder gradually. When the mixture becomes so thick that you can no longer stir it with a spoon, pour it out into a large bowl and knead in the rest of the protein powder. When the ball is of consistent texture, cut it in half and press out one half in each of the two prepared baking pans.

Refrigerate the bar mixture for a half hour to an hour or until it becomes more firm. Cut the bars in thirds in one direction, then in eighths the other direction. (Result: 24 bars per pan.) Roll each bar in the combined topping ingredients:

1 tablespoon finely ground coffee

3 tablespoons ground flax seed

2 tablespoons organic sugar

Store the bars in a tightly sealed container in the refrigerator. They will keep well for one week.

One serving (3 bars) contains 9 grams of protein, 4.8 grams of fat, 20 grams of carboydrate and 150 calories. I find that three of them keep my energy high through late morning.

THE BASIC SMOOTHIE

1 apple quartered and cored

1 orange peeled, cut in half to reveal seeds
   Pull out the seeds.

1 cup of apple juice

2 scoops of protein powder (Use whatever amount is
   recommended on the package as "a serving.")

1 tablespoon of flaxseed oil (omega-3 oil)

1/4 teaspoon of powdered vitamin C (optional, but great
for the immune system)

Blend. Makes approximately 24 ounces. Can be modified with whatever you have on hand. Throw in a piece of fruit that's getting too ripe, and it will add a wonderful and different flavor. Or throw in a few frozen strawberries, blueberries, raspberries or cranberries, and it will taste and look different. Throw in half a banana, and it will be much creamier, as well as now having a taste of banana. My husband and I usually split this if he's home in the morning. Otherwise I drink it all myself.

As you can see, this smoothie gives you a good start on both your fresh fruit and protein requirements.

COOKING BEANS AND SOUPS

There are two things I could not do without in my kitchen. One is my *Le Creuset* enameled cast-iron Dutch oven that I use endlessly for cooking beans. The other is my Farberware® soup kettle. You will see many recipes below that would not turn out so well if I did not own these two pots. I use both of them at least once a week. The Farberware soup kettle is also often used for steaming vegetables with a little stainless steel fold-up steaming baskets.

With the information currently available on the correlation between Alzheimer's and aluminum, I don't think that cooking in aluminum cookware makes sense. Nor do I think that it makes sense to cook in nonstick pots and pans that have been scratched so that those exotic chemicals, whatever they are, are chipping off into the food. The better cookware has nonstick surfaces that don't scratch and chip, which is a much better idea in terms of protecting your health.

MINESTRONE SOUP

2 tablespoons of olive oil

1 large onion, chopped

2 ribs of celery, chopped

4 cloves of fresh garlic, finely chopped or squeezed through a garlic press

6 cups of broth. (I like vegetarian broth, but chicken broth can also be used.)

2 teaspoons of dried basil

2 large scraped carrots, chopped

2 zucchini, or half of a winter squash, depending on the season

8 ounces of the uncooked pasta of your choice (I like penne pasta.)

3 to 6 cups of cooked kidney beans

Sauté the onion, celery and garlic in olive oil. When the onion is translucent, add broth, basil and carrots. Bring to a boil, then turn heat down to a simmer. In 10 minutes, add the zucchini or squash. Cook another 10 minutes, and then add the uncooked pasta. Just before serving, add the beans. Heat long enough to make sure the beans are hot. Serve with grated Parmesan and lots of cracked pepper.

GREEK LIMA BEANS

This came from a friend of a friend. These beans have a unique taste. When they are done, you wouldn't know they were lima beans.

1 pound of dried lima beans
4 tablespoons of olive oil
2 tomatoes, skinned and chopped
a small can of tomato sauce
3-4 cloves of garlic, chopped
2 large carrots, chopped
2 large onions, chopped

After sorting and rinsing the limas, cover them with water, bring to boil, then drain off the water. Refill with water. Bring to a boil and skim the foam over the next 15 minutes or so. Gradually turn the heat down as the foam dissipates. Add the other ingredients. Cook for another hour or so on very low heat, stirring occasionally to make sure the ingredients don't stick to the pot. Makes approximately 12 cups of beans.

BLACK BEAN SOUP

1 pound of dried black beans
4 tablespoons of olive oil
2 onions, chopped
2 green peppers, cored and chopped

6 cloves of garlic, pressed or finely minced
4 cups of vegetable stock
1 teaspoon of cumin
1 teaspoon of oregano
2 tablespoons of vinegar

Sort, rinse and cook the beans in water in a heavy bean pot, skimming off the foam as it appears on the surface. When the beans are cooked, in a separate kettle, sauté the onions, green pepper and garlic in oil. When the onions are translucent, add the beans, broth and remaining ingredients to the soup kettle. Cook at least a half hour, though longer is better if you have the time. Makes approximately 16 cups of soup.

SALAD DRESSINGS/VEGGIE DIP

Here are two salad dressings you can make at home. This can help you avoid store-bought bottled dressings that are loaded with additives. The second recipe doubles as a vegetable dip.

LYNN'S SALAD DRESSING

4 huge cloves of garlic, pressed or finely minced
1 1/2 teaspoon of Dijon mustard
the juice of one-half of a lemon
2/3 cup of olive oil
1/3 cup of cider vinegar
a teaspoon of Worchester sauce

Combine the ingredients in a jar that has a good lid.

Then close it and shake the mixture well. This dressing is better after a couple of days, as the garlic has a chance to permeate the liquids. It's a very healthful salad dressing. If you don't want the calories or fat of spooning it liberally over your salad, squeeze half a lemon over your salad, and have the dressing on the side in a small finger-type bowl. Dip each biteful of salad lightly in the dressing. Makes 1+ cup of dressing.

KATE'S SALAD DRESSING & VEGGIE DIP

1/3 cup of Bragg's liquid aminos
1/3 cup of lemon juice
1/3 cup of water
2 cups of raw sesame seeds

Add to taste:
Salt
Pepper
Ginger
Red pepper (optional)
Parsley or cilantro

Put the first three ingredients in a blender. With the blender on, gradually add raw sesame seeds until the mixture just begins to thicken. Adjust flavor with salt or salt substitute, pepper, ginger and red pepper (if desired) to taste. Then add parsley or cilantro until the dressing/dip is thickened. Makes 3 cups.

YOGURT DIP FOR VEGGIE

1 cup of yogurt
juice of 1/2 lemon
1/2 teaspoon of dill seed
fresh ground pepper to taste.
dash of Worcestershire sauce
1 teaspoon of sugar

POPCORN SPRAY
(also good on steamed veggies or potatoes)

1/4 cup of olive oil
2 tablespoons of Braggs Liquid Amino Acids
1/2 teaspoon of garlic juice, available from health food
  store

Mix well, then pour into a spray bottle.

A DETOX SOUP

1 1/2 onions
3 ribs of celery
6 cloves of garlic
10 cups of vegetable broth
8 medium carrots (5 large), sliced thinly
1 28-ounce can of tomatoes
1/4 head of cabbage, slices thinly
2 zucchini, sliced
1 bunch of chard, sliced into strips across the leaf
2 tablespoons of basil

1 tablespoon of oregano
1 winter squash (such as butternut or spaghetti squash)

Chop the onions, celery and garlic and place in a large, heavy-bottomed soup pot. Spray these vegetables with an all-natural vegetable oil pan coating (available from a health food store). Sauté over very low heat, stirring frequently, until the onions and celery wilt. Then add broth, bring to a boil, turn down heat and add remaining ingredients. Simmer until all ingredients are tender, about 30 minutes. This recipe does not have to be followed exactly. Though it's much better to use organic vegetables when you're detoxing, it's also good to use up what you have in the vegetable bin. Makes approximately 20 cups of soup. It can also be used to produce delicious vegetable broth. Just strain out the broth and save the vegetables to eat by themselves or with rice at another time.

HOW TO COOK BROWN RICE

Rice is very important to detox diets because it's much more easily digested than other grains. Also, many people are allergic to wheat and don't know it.

While both white rice and brown rice are very nutritious, brown rice offers a lot of fiber and more flavor. On the other hand, because brown rice retains some of the natural oils of the grain, it can go rancid after a few months in storage. Avoid this problem by storing the brown rice in the refrigerator.

Ingesting rancid oils raises the level of harmful free-radicals and oxidative stress in the bloodstream. If you find brown rice has acquired a strange and not altogether pleasant odor, it's best to compost it or throw it away.

The following is a foolproof method for cooking brown rice, courtesy of Annette Annechild.

Either:

2 1/3 cups of rice to 4 cups of water, or

3 1/2 cups of rice to 6 cups of water

Rinse the uncooked rice three times and drain well. Put the water on to boil in a cooking pot. While waiting for the water to come to a boil, put two tablespoons of oil in the bottom of a heavy, tight-lidded saucepan. Sauté the well-drained rice in the oil for approximately four minutes while you wait for the water to boil. Do this over fairly high heat. It has to be stirred constantly, otherwise it will scorch. This process coats the rice with the oil and evaporates the water from rinsing. The rice will begin to smell very nutty after a minute or two.

When the water pot has come to a vigorous boil, pour it over the rice in the saucepan. It is very important at this point not to stir the rice anymore, not even once. Let the liquid come back up to a vigorous boil, put the lid on, turn the heat down as low as you can, and cook this for 45 minutes. (The cooking temperature is different on a electric stove. The lowest setting will be too low. You may have to experiment on your own stove to determine the correct temperature.) During this time, do not lift the lid or do anything else to it. After 45 minutes, turn off the heat and let the rice sit undisturbed for at least 15-20 minutes before serving.

The result? Healthy, delicious and nicely textured rice.

INDEX

1997 Guide to Yoga Teachers & Classes, 277

7-Day Detox Miracle, 158, 256, 299

A

acetaminophen, 242

Achilea millefolium, 162

acid/alkaline balance, 161

acupressure, 289

acupuncture, 289

addiction, 24, 254

adenosine triphosphate, 106

adrenal glands, 64

stimulated by saunas and showers, 299

adrenaline, 40

overload, 47

aerobic exercise, 276

affirmations, 110

age spots, prevention, and dandelion, 272

aging, detox for slowing , 272

air pollution, 259

alcohol, 19, 254

aldehydes, 244

Aleve, 242

Alka Gold, 245

Alka Seltzer, 245

alkaline, 161

All Bran, for regularity, 264

Allen, David, 112

allergens, 108

allergic, 227

Alllium sativum, 271

almond oil, 143

alpha-linolenic acids, 127, 130

alternative medicine, bodywork as most popular form, 286

Alzheimer's disease, 195

amaryllis, 137

Amer. Massage Therapy Ass'n, 290

amino acids, 168; antioxidant , 255; necessary for detox, 254

Anatomy of an Illness, 39

anemia, 195; and yellow dock root, 272; and burdock, 271

anger, 109

angina, 195

animal fats, 128

anticipation, 38

antihistamines, 195

antioxidant , 85

antioxidant (as used in marketing), 255

antioxidant vitamins, 159-160, 207, 238, 242; and minerals, 42, 156; characteristic of milk thistle, 270; 4 in green tea, 261

anxiety, 69, 92, 195, 308

appetite suppresant, red clover as, 272

apple (s), 210, 53, 57, 58, 82, 89, 114; for regularity, 264

apple cider vinegar, 160

apple pectin, for regularity, 264

apricot oil, 145

apricots, 53

aquifer, 23

aroma etiquette, 148

aromatherapy, 40, 97, 135, 140, 141-146

arteries, 256

arthritis, 62; rheumatoid, 287

arugula, 228

Asian foods, 101

aspirin, 242, 245

asthma, 195; bronchial, 76

autoimmune condition, 192

autonomic nervous system, 291

avocado (s), 214, 301

Ayurvedic Concepts, 244

Ayurvedic remedy, 244

Ayurvedic tradition for inducing perspiration, 296

B

B vitamins, 167

babaganooj, 123
back bends, 281
back problems, 62, 105
back stretch, 171
bacteria, 75, 108; and immune
    system, 272; saunas and immune
    system, 299
bacterial waste products, 254
bad breath, 42
baked products, commercial, 128
Baker, Sidney MacDonald Baker,
    M.D., 80-83, 127, 167, 254
baking, 129
baking soda, 161, 245
balance postures, 281
Balch, James F., M.D., 166
Balch, Phyllis A., C.N.C., 166
ballet, 38, 69
banana (s), 57; as potassium
    replacement, 298
barbeque, 218, 225
Barrie, Stephen, N.D., 158, 256, 299
bartending, 113
bath (s), hot, 187; public, 156; sponge,
    71
bathing , 40, 153-163; detox, 155;
therapeutic, 156
bathroom, 135, 153-156
bean soup, homemade, 82
bean spread, 120
beans, garbanzo, 123; pinto, refried,
    120
Beattie, Melanie, 25
beauty treatment, 177
beef, 84
beer, 19, 126
beet juice, 212, 238
behaviorism, 29
bellows breath, 106
Bennett, Peter, N.D., 158, 256, 299
bentonite clay, 244
benzodiazepines, 191
Berra, Yogi, 109
berries, 59
beta carotene, 167
betacarotine, as an antioxidant, 255
Bible, 142
Bifido Factor, 244
Bifidobacterium bifidum, 244
bike, stationary, 68

bile, and milk thistle, 270; as it relates
    to detox, 257
bile duct, 257
binge/purge dynamic, 266
biochemical issues, 165
bioflavonoids, 167; antioxidant, 255
biotin, 168
birch oil, 146
birds, 52
bird-watching, 65
Blackjack, 17-18
bladder, overactive, 194
Bland, Jeffrey, Ph.D., 166, 256, 272
blessed thistle (*Cerbenia benedicta*), 162
blood, 41, 75
blood alcohol level, 178, 240
blood pressure reduction, via t'ai chi,
    283; high, and saunas, 297
blood purifier, red clover as, 272;
    yellow dock root as, 272
blood vessels, 64
blood, role in detoxification, 256
body temperature, 187
*Body: What Type of Massage to Get
    and How to Make the Most of It*, 288
bodywork and massage, 285-294
boneset (Eupatorium perfoliatum),
    162
Bonham, John, 187
boundaries, 93
bourbon, 241
bowel cleansing kits, 262
bowels, 41; role in detoxification, 255
Bragg's Amino Acids, 125, 231, 263,
brain cells, 62
brain-washing, 183
brandy, 241
bread, 100, 136; with butter, 228;
homemade, 200
breast cancer, 85
breath, in yoga, 276
breathing, 77
breathing break, 107
brown bag lunch, 91, 98
brown rice fast, 263
building techniques, conventional,
    259
burdock root (Arctium lappa), 271
burn-out, 23
burrito, 230

butter, 128

C

cabbage, 211; red, 211, 214
caffeine, 19, 64, 79, 190; relative to
    detox, 260
caffeine withdrawal headache, 261,
    268
calcium, 166, 168, 169
calcium citrate, 168, 191
Calistoga Spa Hot Springs, 305
cancer, 28, 42, 62, 131; formation,
    130; prevention, 59; rates,
    268; and garlic, 271; breast, and
    dandelion, 272
cancer-causing, 100
candlelight, 133-135, 139-140
candles, 139,185; nontoxic, 140;
    scented, 140
candy, hard, 124
capillaries, 75, 256
carbohydrates, 79, 81, 82, 83, 100,
    216
carbon dioxide, 256
carbonated drinks, 261
carbonation, 241
cardiovascular disease, 84
career pressures, 95
carnations, 136
carpets, new, 108
carrier oil, 143
carrot (s), 211; juice, 238; sticks, 69,
    124; baby, 124
cascara sagrada (*Rhamnus purshiana*),
    263
catnip (*Nepata cataria*), 162, 191
cedarwood oil, 143
celery, 124, 211, 214
cell membranes, 128
cell metabolism, as it relates to detox,
    257
cells, dead, 75; mutated, 130
cellular material, 254
central nervous system, 291
ceramic rings, 143
cereal, dry, 136; high fiber, for
    regularity, 264
chamomile (*Anthemis nobilis*), 144
chamomile (*Matricaria chamomilla*),
    162, 190

champagne, 241, 242
chardonnays, 248
cheeks, rosy, 64
cheese, 84, 249
chemical exposure, 156; and saunas,
    297
chemically sensitive, 140, 147
chemicals, 42; industrial, 158
chemotherapy, 76
cherimoya, 55
cherries, 53, 59
chi, Chinese term for lifeforce, 276
chicken, 84
child's pose, 172
chime, wake-up, 47
Chinese cuisine, 131
chips 121
chiropractors, 287, 290
chocolate, 19, 69, 128, 190; chips, 69;
    hot, 190
cholesterol-lowering claims, 87
choline, 168
Chopra Center for Well-Being, 138
chronic conditions, detox for
    reversing, 272
chronic illness, bodywork for, 286
chronic obstructive pulmonary
    disease, 195
chronobiology, 81
chronopharmacology, 81
cinnamon (*Cinnamomum zeylanicum*),
    150
cinnamon, essential oil, 77, 145; tea,
    193
circadian, 80
Circadian Prescription, The, 80, 83
circadian rhythms, 184
circulation, 36, 41, 64; system, 169; to
    digestive system, and saunas, 299;
    improvement via saunas, 298;
    improvement via t'ai chi, 284;
    stimulated by salt rub, 301
circulatory system, role in
    detoxification, 256
citrus, 265; oil, 58, 143, 145, 148
Claire, Thomas, 288-289
clary sage (*Salvia sclarea*), 150
cleaner, nontoxic, 159
Cleopatra, 142
clock (s), 47, 186; alarm, 47, 184;
    Zen, 47

clove oil, 301
cobalamin, 167
Coca-Cola, 245
cocaine, 254
coconut, 126; oil, 128
Codependent No More, 25
coffee, 19, 68, 79, 101, 190, 249; grinder, 102; shop, 228; Irish, 242
cognitive ability, 183
cold shower following sauna, 298
collagen, 74
colon, 130; function and yellow dock root, 272
colonics, 262
community-supported agriculture, 201-203
complexion, poor, 42
concentration, 276
conflict resolution, 96, 111
Cong Fou of the Tao-Tse, 287
congeners, 241
congestion, reduced by saunas and showers, 299
consciousness, 136
constipation, 130; chronic, 264
conversation, 135
cookies, 249
Cooperative Extension, 203
copper (gluconate), 168
corn oil, 127
corn tortilla, 119
corn-based cuisine, 227
coronary artery disease, 195
coronary heart disease, 131
cottage cheese, 123
cottonseed oil, 127
coughs, red clover for, 272
County Department of Mental Healthcare, 196
cow's milk, 130
cranberries, 211
cranberry/raspberry juice, 102
cravings, 83
creativity, 98
cucumber, 212, 214, 302
curly dock, 272
cypress *(Cypressus sempervirens)*, 150
cypress oil, 146

D
dairy, 19, 84, 259, 261, 267

dairy-free, 232
dancing, 240; classes, 67; after drinking, 243
dandelion *(Taraxacum officinale)*, 271
dandelion tea, 239
day spa, 304-305
daylight, 184
De Sanitate Tuenda, 285
deep breathing, 40
degenerative disease, 61
dehydrogenase, 245
deli foods, 215; Italian, 247
delicatessen, 228
depression, 42, 62, 191, 195
deprivation, 134; avoiding while detoxing, 266
Desert Hot Springs Spa Hotel, 305
designated driver, 240
dessert, 58
detox, 36, 188, 253-273; baths, 245; tea, 102; and home spa techniques, 300; personal, 158
detoxification, 42, 58, 60, 74, 128, 158, 162, 166, 169; medically supervised, 254; enhanced by saunas and showers, 299; role of skin in, 295
Detoxification & Healing: The Key to Optimal Health, 127, 167, 254
diabetes, 28, 41, 62, 131, 216
diabetic, 227; caution re reflexology for, 291
diet, 42; low-carbohydrate, 225
dietary preferences, 19
digestion, 58, 66, 81, 83; related to detox, 257
digestive juices, 81
dioxins, 100
disharmony, 138
diuretic, use of dandelion as, 271
doctor, 62
downshifting, 133
dreams, vivid, 192
drowsiness, 178, 195
drug store, 72
drumbeat, 138
dry skin masque, 301; brushing, 42, 72, 74, 76
E
earplugs, 193, 236
echinacea *(Echinacea angustifolia)*, 272

e-coli, 84
ecosystem, 23
Edwards, Rem B., 27
egg whites, 301
eggplant, 123, 204
eggs, 82
Egyptions, ancient, 142
Ehret, Charles, Dr., 80
Einstein, Albert, 183
elastin, 74
emotion, 142
emotional issues, 165; bodywork for, 286
emotional uneasiness, while detoxing, 264
emotions, suppressed, 40
employees, high-tech, 79
endocrine system, stimulated by saunas and showers, 299
endorphins, released by bodywork, 286
endotoxins, 254, 258
enemas, 262
energy, 41, 79, 83, 165, 190
energy bars, commercial, 99; homemade, 82, 86, 99
energy pulsation, rhythmic, 277
energy, vital, 276
enjoyment, 37
enkephalins, released by bodywork, 286
entrainment, 138
epidemiological studies, 85, 130
Epsom salts, 158, 160
ergonomics, 105
essential fatty acids, 127-129
essential oils, 77, 140, 141
estrogen replacement, 85
eucalyptus (*Eucalyptus globulus*), 150, 300
eucalyptus oil, 145
evening primrose oil, 238
evolution, 61, 81
Excedrin, 242
excretion, 41
exercise, 20, 41, 76, 156, 186, 268; lack of, 42
exfoliation, 74, 159; via salt rub, 301
exotoxins, 254, 258
extravagance, 136

eye treatments and facial masques, 302-303
eye-hand coordination, 69

F
facial masques, 302
fajitas, 226
familial strength, 135
family dinner, 134
farm workers, 53
farmers' market, 200
fast food, 100
fat, 216
fat, beef, 230
fatigue, 42, 156, 182; while traveling, 233
fatty acid deficiencies, 128
FDA, 87
feet, cold, 187
feet, relating to reflexology, 288-294
fermentation, 241
fertilizers, 259
fiber, as it relates to detox, 257; as it relates to regularity, 263
final relaxation, 281
fish, 84, 225, 267; oil, 127; grilled, 82
fitness, ugly duckling of, 61
flatulence, 120
flaxseed oil, 56, 127, 129, 130, 238
flaxseeds, organic, 130
flight or fight syndrome, 40
flowers, 97, 133-137, 141, 200
flu-like symptoms, 147
folic acid, 168
food, 108; budgets, 215; combining, 81, 100; courts, 232; protein-dense, 190; quality, 36; safety, 84
food stores, specialty, 247
footmaps, Chinese and Egyptian, 289
forest, 49, 141
forward bend, 104, 281
fountain, 98
frankincense (*Boswellia thurifera*), 142, 145, 150
frankincense oil, 148
free radical, 255
freedom, 183
French fries, 230
French press, 102
fried foods, 128
Frontier Bombay Veggie Blend, 123

frozen foods, 215
fruit (s), 99, 243, 82; juice, fresh, 82; pudding, 209, 213; juice bars, frozen, 126; tropical, 210
fruits and vegetables, fresh, 42, 59, 124, 156, 216, 238; for fasting, 264; in how to detox, 258
fuel pump, 36
fumigants, 158
furniture, new, 108

G
gait problems, 62
Galen, 285
gall bladder and yellow dock root, 272; and burdock root, 271
gardening, 37; container, 137
garlic (*Alllium sativum*), 123, 125,168, 227, 239, 271; juice, 125; odor-less, 239
gas pedal, 35
Gattefosse, Rene-Maurice, 142
genetics, 269
geranium (*Pelargonium graveolens*), 150
geranium oil, 145
Getting Things Done, The Art of Stress-Free Productivity, 112
gin, 241
ginger (*Zingiber officinale*), 125, 150, 162, 212, 238; oil, 145; tea, 245
ginkgo biloba, 168
Glen Ivy, 305
glucose, 182, 192
glutamine, 211
glutatione, as an antioxidant, 255; from milk thistle, 270
gluten, 227
gluten-free, 232
glycogen, 106
goals, 96
goat's milk, 130
gold, 142
golf, 29, 220
Gone with the Wind, 238
gourmet store, 247
gout, and burdock root, 271
granola, 100
grapefruit, 53
grapefruit (*Citrus paradisi*), 150; essential oil, 77; juice, 210

grapes, 53, 124, 214, 243; as a monofast, 265
greasy foods, 245
Greek cuisine, 131; restaurants, 123
green tea, 261
Greer, Rosy, 186
grocers, 53
grocery, Japanese, 247
grooming, 154
ground beef, 87
guacamole, 226
guava, 55
gym, 67, 69, 71

H
Haas, Elson M., M.D., 166
hair of the dog, 245
hairdos, 182
Halls' Sugar-Free Mentholyptus Cough Drops, 193
hamburgers, 100
hangover, 238, 239
happiness, 39
Harvey, William, 287
headache (s), 147; remedy, 242; while detoxing, 264, 269
headphone or headset, 106, 139, 221, 292
health department regulations, 218
health food store, 72, 77, 86, 87, 115, 124, 125, 130, 169, 191, 212, 213, 239, 244, 262, 264
health, emotional, 38
healthcare educators, 28
healthcare, insightful, 20
HealthComm International, 272
heart, 75
heart disease, 28, 41, 61, 84; and saunas, 297; prevention, 59
heart problems, major, 76
heart rate, lowering via t'ai chi, 283
heat and inflammation, 299
herb tea, 190; detox, 42
herbal extract, 270
herbal medicine, 269
herbalists, 269
herbicides, 259
herbs, 168
Herbs for Detoxification, 266
heroin, 254

hierarchy of needs, 108
high blood pressure, 129, 158; and saunas, 297
Hippocrates, 285
Hobbs, Christopher, L.Ac., 166
holistic healthcare, 19
holistic practitioners, 18, 19, 158
honey, 200
hops (*Hummulus lupulus*), 191
hormonal fluctuations, 179
hormonal issues, 165
hormones, 254; prostanoid, 127
hors d'oeuvre, 124, 126, 204
horsetail (Equisetum arvense), 162
hot flashes, 85, 187
hot springs, 305
hot sweats, 194
hot tubs, 156
hot water bottle, 187
hummus, 123
hunger, 83
Huygens, Christian, 138
hydration while drinking, 239
hydrogen peroxide, 160, 161
hydrogenated oils, 128
hypertension, 195
hypoglycemic, 119

I
ibuprofen, 242
Ice Age, 40
immortality, 20
immune stimulant, echinacea as, 272
immune support, 59
immune system, 38, 39, 138, 178, 209; response, 155; and burdock root, 271; and garlic, 271; saunas and, 299
immunity enhancement, via t'ai chi, 284
incandescent bulbs, 139
incense, 248
India, 248, 275
Indian cuisine, 131
Indian spiritual masters, 277
indigestion, 58, 188
individuality, 183
indoor air quality, 107
indulgences, 259

infectious agents and immune system, 272
inflammation, acute, 76; bodywork for, 286; cold showers and, 299
insomnia, 179
insomniacs, 184
instinctual behavior, 183
insulin resistance, 179
insurance companies, 285
internal tissue detoxification, 155
interstitial fluid, 256
intestines, role in detoxification, 256
investment banks, 40
ions, negative, 98
ipriflavone, 85
iris, 136
iron, 125
iron absorption, and burdock root, 271
irregular heartbeat, 195
isoflavones, 85, 86
Italian cuisine, 131
Iyengar yoga, 280

J
Japanese-American, 85
jasmine (*Jasminum grandiflorum*), 150
jellyfish, warm, feeling from sauna, 298; from yoga, 277
jerk sauce, 124
Jesuit School of Theology at Berkeley, 249
Jesus, 142
jet lag, 192
jicama, 126
joie de vivre, 276
joint problems, 62
joint stiffness, bodywork for, 286
joints, sore, 146
journal, 174
journal writing, 165
joy, 37
juice bar, 115, 209; fasting, 266; bottled, 209
juicer, citrus, 210
juicers, 212-213
juicing, 42, 207-214, 243
jumping rope, 68
juniper (*Juniperus communis*), 150
juniper berry essential oil, 77, 146

K

karate, 282
kettle, electric, 102
ki, Japanese term for lifeforce, 276
kidney function, and burdock, 271
kidney problems, 76
kidneys, 41, 72; role in detoxification, 255, 256
knitting, 185-186
Kripalu Center, 277
kung fu, 282

L

Lactobacillus acidophilus, 100
large intestine, as it relates to detox, 257
laundry products, 259
Laval University, 184
lavender (*Lavendula officinalis*), 142, 144, 150, 162, 300
lavender oil, 145, 146, 148, 245, 301
lavender shampoo, 146
laxatives, over-the-counter, 264
l-cysteine, 168
lead wires, 140
lemon, 243; balm (*Melissa officinalis*), 191; essential oil, 77; oil, 148; verbena, 146; wedges, 228
lemon juice, 103, 123, 190; as liver cleanser, 272
lethargy, 42; bodywork to reverse, 286
lettuce, 213
l-glutathione, 168
lifeforce, 276
light, artificial, 185; book, 185; brightening, 49
light-headedness while detoxing, 265
lighting, florescent, 139; overhead, 139; table, 139
lightness, 161
lilies, 136
limbic system, 142
lime essential oil, 77; juice, 126
Ling, Per Heinrik, 287
linolenic acids, 127
linseed oil, 127
Liv 52, 244
liver, 169, 182, 187, 188, 240, 245, 263; cleanser, 193; diseases, 270; function and yellow dock root, 272; function, improved by saunas and showers, 299; tonic, use of dandelion as, 271; transplant, 36; and burdock root, 271; and milk thistle, 270
Liver Care, 244
LiveRx, 244
l-methionine, 168
Loma Linda University, 85
loofa sponge, 159
Los Angeles Rams, 186
Los Angeles Times, 268
low density lipoprotein (LDL), 85
lunch, 98-101; packing, 182
lungs, 72, 74; role in detoxification, 256, 257
Lyman, Howard, 259
lymph angions, 75; cleanser, echinacea as, 272; nodes, 75; system, 67, 72, 74, 169
lymph system, bodywork and sauna, 298
lymphatic fluid, 41, 75, 76
lymphatic, initial, 75
lymphocytes, 75

M

mad cow disease, 84
Mad Cowboy, 259
magnesium, 168, 169, 191
manganese (gluconate), 168
mango (es), 53, 55, 126
mango, Manila, 54
mantra, 175
margaritas, 242
marine plant oils, 127
marjoram (*Marjorana hortensis*), 144, 150
Mark Anthony, 142
martial arts, 282
Maslow, Abraham, 108
massage, 40, 42, 76; and bodywork, 285-294; therapist (s), 290, 306; after sauna, 298; Swedish, 287
Master Gardeners, 203
mattress, 193
mayonnaise, 301
McDonald's, 230
McGee-Cooper, Ann, 112

meat, 19, 100, 259, 267
meat (s), grilled, 82
medication (s), 76, 179; over-the-counter, 190; prescription,190
medicine, complementary, Swedish massage as, 288
meditation, 40, 48, 165, 174
Mediterranean climate, 52; diet, 130
melatonin, 192
Melita filter, 102
melon (s), 53, 58
menopause, 85, 194
mental clarity, 161
meridians, 275
metabolic processes, in how to detox, 257
Metabolic Response Modifiers, 244
metabolic waste and saunas, 299
Mexican food, 230
microwave chipmaker, 121
Middle Eastern restaurants, 123
milk thistle (*Silybum marianum*), 168, 239, 263, 270
mind, conscious, 141
    unconscious, 141
mineral content, 217
minerals, 168, 207; antioxidant, 255; necessary for detox, 254
mint, 300
miscarriage, potential for, 291
mitochondria, 106
moderate behavior, 247
mold (s), 108, 209
molybdenum, 168
Montreal Canadiens, 186
Moon, Keith, 187
morning news, 184
Mother Nature, 141
Motrin, 242
muscle relaxants, 169
muscles, stiff, 169
mushrooms, poisonous, 270
music, 63, 97, 116, 134, 135; classical, 97
musicians, 200
myrrh (*Commiphora myrrha*), 142, 150

N
nap, as hangover remedy, 245
Napa Valley, 305

nasal congestion, 195
National Sleep Foundation, 179
Native American sweat lodges, 296
nativity story, 142
Natren, 244
Natural Liver Therapy, 166
nature sounds, 48
naturopathic physician (s), 79, 269
nausea, 147, 245; while detoxing, 264, 269
necklaces (for essential oils), 143
nervous system, 38
neurotoxins, 147
New England Journal of Medicine, 85
New York Yankees, 109
NFL Hall of Fame, 186
niacin, 167
niacinamide, 167
non-impact activity, t'ai chi as, 283
Norman Cousins, 39
Norman, Laura, 294
nutrients, 42
nutritional supplements, 20, 166, 268
nutritionist, 169
nuts, 200

O
oatmeal as facial masque, 301; for regularity, 264
oatstraw, 162
obesity, 28, 216
obstructive sleep apnea, 195
ofuros, 156
oil change (analogy for detox), 253; filter, 36; glands, 74; pump, 36
olive oil, 125, 188, 231, 238
olive, black, paste, 204
Omega 3 oil, 56
omega-3 fatty acid, 127
omega-6 fatty acid, 127
onions, 214; green, 214
opposable thumb & forefinger, 289
orange (s) (*Citrus sinensis*), 53, 58, 150, 210, 211; juice, 207, 210; peel, 190; blood, 55
orange bergamot essential oil, 77
orchid, 137
organ function, improved by saunas and showers, 299
organic foods, 156; while detoxing, 265

organizational techniques, 96
organizer, 174
organizing systems, 112
orthopedic surgeons, 63
oscillators, 138
osmosis, 161
osteoporosis, 62, 85; prevention via
    t'ai chi, 284
outcomes, successful, 96
outgassing, 259
overwhemed, 39
oxidation, 208, 255
oxidative stress relative to detox, 269;
    while detoxing, 265
oxygen, 108, 160; as it relates to
    detox, 256

P
pain and inflammation, 299
pain killers, 169, 254
pain relief, bodywork for, 286; yoga
    for, 276
palm kernel oil, 128
pancreas, 257; function and
    dandelion, 272
panic, 109
pantothenic acid, 167
papayas, 55
parenting, 177
Parkinson's disease, 195
Parmesan cheese, 125
Parnell, Devakanya, G., 277
parsley, 211
passionflower (*Passiflora incarnata*),
    191
passionfruit, 55, 211
pasta, 82
pasteurization, 208
pastries, 249
peach (es), 51, 53
peanut oil, 127
peanut-butter, 124
pear, 58
pecans, 214
Pellegrino, 240
peppermint (*Mentha piperita*), 150
peppermint (*Mentha pulegium*), 162;
    oil, 77, 145; tea, 302
perfume, 133, 147
perfume making, 145

perimenopause, 179
persimmons, 53
personal care products, 141, 145, 259
personalities, difficult, 96
perspiration, 72
pesticides, 259
petrochemicals, 72, 140
pharmacist, 190
photography, 66, 67
physiatrist, 62
physical activity, 186
physical education classes, 69
physical therapist, 62, 63
physician, naturopathic, 79
phytonutrients, 52, 207
picnic, 204
Pilates-based training, 69
pine (*Pinus species*), 150
pine essential oil, 77, 145, 148
pineapple, 210, 211, 243
planned-overs, 100, 217
Plante, Jacques, 186
plum, elephant heart, 55
plums, 53, 265
plywood, 259
PMS, 179
poetry, 70
pollutants, 108
pomegranates, 53
popcorn, air-popped, 125
pores, 74
positive stimulation, 35
posture problems, 62
postures, inverted, in yoga, 281
potassium, 168, 240; loss during
    sauna, 298
potato, baked, 188, 231, 245, 255
potatoes, 82
poultry, 267; grilled, 82
Poutinen, C. J., 266
prana, Indian term for lifeforce, 275,
    276
prayer, 70
prayer walking, 70
pregnancy, 76, 179; caution re saunas,
    297; caution re reflexology, 291
pregnant, 143, 158
Prescription for Nutritional Healing,
    166
prescription glasses, 105

prescription tranquilizers, 254
preservatives, 216, 217
presswood, 259
pretzels, 124
preventive health care, 18, 216
probiotics, 100
produce stands, 54
progressive relaxation, 189
props, in yoga, 280
prostate cancer, 85
prostate problems, 194
protein, 75, 79, 81, 83, 100, 268; bar(s), 82, 86, 89, 114, 231, 238; powder, 56, 169; excess, 76
psychoneuroimmunology, 38
psyllium husk, 264
public relations, 113
public transportation, 148
pumpkin seeds, 100
pycnogenol, 168
pyridoxine, 167

R
radishes, 211, 213
reading, 185
rebounder, 67
red clover (*Trifolium pratense*), 272
redness and inflammation, 299
reflex spots, 288
reflexologist, professional, 294
reflexology, 288-294; hand, 291-292
relationship building, 66
relationships, problem, 39
relaxant, red clover as, 272
relaxation, 154; in yoga, 276
Renaissance artists, 52
repressive regimes, 183
resentment, 109
respiratory specific, red clover as, 272
restaurant (s), 113; ethnic, 225-228, 238; meals, 215
rheumatoid arthritis, 287
rhythmic breathing, in yoga, 276
riboflavin, 167
rice , 245; bread, 262; brown, 238; cake, 123; cereals, 262; in detox, 262; pasta, 19, 262; plain white, to slow detox, 267
rice, brown, 238; as a fast, 263; in regularity, 263
rice-based, 227

Rider, Mark, Ph.D., 137
right-fat foods, 216; snacks, 41
rock stars, 187
rollerblading, 30
romaine, 228
Romans, 259
romantic, 133
room temperature, 187
roots, 141
rose, 97, 136, oil (*Rosa damascena*), 146, 148. 150; petal, 148
rosemary essential oil, 77
Royal Institute of Gymnastics, 287
rum, 241

S
sad dock, 272
salad (s), 58, 82, 101, 249; bar, 238; Chef's, 229; European-type, 228
salad dressing (s), 129, 229
salmonella, 84
salsa, 120, 121, 226, 231
salt, 217
sandalwood (*Santalum album*), 150
sandwiches, 100
sarsaparilla (*Smilax ornata*), 272
saturated fat (s), 100, 128, 225
sauna (s), 40, 42, 69, 245, 295-300; Finnish style, 296; and pregnancy cautions, 297
sauna therapists, 297
sausages, 249
scent, 134; characteristic, 141; coordinated products, 146
scotch, 241
sea salt, 161
seeds, 141
selenium, 168; as an antioxidant, 255
self-actualization, 108
self-improvement experts, 110
self-soothing, 186
senna (*Cassia acutifolia*), 263
serum insulin levels, high, 81
sesame oil, 143, 145
Seventh-Day Adventitst, 85
Shakespeare, 177
shallots, 214
shamanistic traditions, 138
shampoo, fragrance-free, 77, 145
Sharp Cabrillo Hospital, 138

sherbet, 209, 213
sherry, 241
shower, cold, following sauna, 298
showers, hot, 71, 117
Silybum marianum, 263
silymarin, 168
Simon, David, MD, 138
sisal mitt, 159
skin, 41, 72; disorders and yellow
    dock root, 272; treatments at day
    spas, 305; exercising the, 74;
    related to detoxification, 295
skullcap *(Scutellaria laterifolia)*, 191
sleep, 177-196; deep, 183; deprivation,
    183; hygiene, 139, 182, 184-193;
    medications, over-the-counter, 195;
    REM, 183
sleeping problems, 92
small intestine, as it relates to detox,
    257
smog, 40
smoking, 20, 193
smoothie (s), 56, 82, 100, 169, 209,
    238, 270
snacking, low-calorie, 119
snacks, right-fat, 119-127
snoring, 192-193
social graces, 135
soda crackers, 245
soft drinks, 190
sorbet, 126, 209, 213
soup, broth-based, 228
soups, 217
soups, homemade, 101
Southern Methodist University, 138
soy, 84-88; milk, 130; nuts, 82, 114,
    124; sauce, 231
soy snack foods, 87-88; comparison
    chart, 88
soybean, 84; oil, 127
spa (s) and spa culture, 295-306;
    activities, 42; at home techniques,
    300-304; backyard, 156; day, 304-
    305; destination, 304; experience,
    40; old, 305
spearmint tea, 302
spices, 248
spicy food, 227
spider plants, 97, 108
Spike; 123; salt-free, 123

spinach, 211
spinal twist (s), 172, 281
spiritual connectedness, 37; masters,
    110; support, 39; tradition, 175
spleen, 76; function and dandelion,
    272; function and yellow dock root,
    272
sports injuries, bodywork for, 286
sprouts, 214
spruce essential oil, 77
stairs, 67
standing forward bend, 170
steak houses, 225
stews, 217
stir-fry, 82
stomach function and dandelion, 272
straps, in yoga, 280
strawberries, 53
strength, 278
stress, 25, 38, 61, 105, 178; as relieved
    by reflexology, 291; hormones, 40,
    259; relief, 106; stress management,
    20, 143; while traveling, 233; yoga
    for, 276, 278
stress reduction, 36, 39, 134, 155; t'ai
    chi for , 283; via bodywork, 286
stretching, 165, 185; in yoga, 276
stroke, 61
subconscious, 110
substance abuse, 254
sugar, 19, 79
Sun Salutation, 281
sunflower seeds, 100, 214, 231
surfing, 95
sustainability, 23, 24
sweat glands, 74
sweat lodges, Native American, 296
Swedish massage, 287
sweet basil essential oil, 77
sweet orange essential oil, 77
sweet peas, 136
sweets, 192
swelling and inflammation, 299
swimming, 67; pools, 156

T
Taco Bell, 230
tahini, 123
t'ai chi, 67, 282-284
tangerine essential oil, 77